PAR. Pseudo-Allergic Reactions, Vol. 4
Idiopathic, Food-Induced and Drug-Induced Pseudo-Allergic Reactions

PAR
Pseudo-Allergic Reactions

Involvement of Drugs and Chemicals

Vol. 4

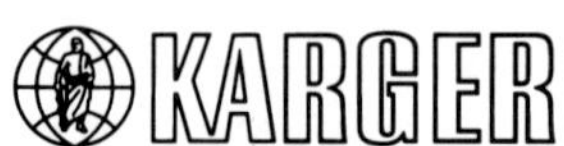

S. Karger · Basel · München · Paris · London · New York · Tokyo · Sydney

Idiopathic, Food-Induced and Drug-Induced Pseudo-Allergic Reactions

Editors
P. Dukor, Basel; P. Kallós, Helsingborg;
H.D. Schlumberger, Wuppertal; G.B. West, Epsom, Surrey

19 figures and 33 tables, 1985

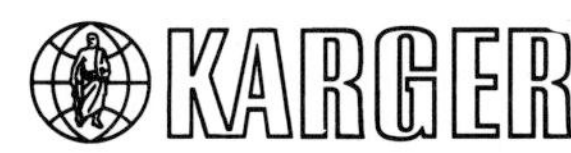

S. Karger · Basel · München · Paris · London · New York · Tokyo · Sydney

PAR. Pseudo-Allergic Reactions

Involvement of Drugs and Chemicals

Dukor, P., Basel; Kallós, P., Helsingborg; Schlumberger, H.D., Wuppertal; West, G.B., Epsom, Surrey (eds.)

Vol. 1: Genetic Aspects and Anaphylactoid Reactions.
XIV + 310 p., 57 fig., 40 tab., 1980. ISBN 3-8055-0537-X

Vol. 2: Cytotoxic and Complement Mediated Reactions.
VIII + 144 p., 21 fig., 20 tab., 1980. ISBN 3-8055-0666-X

Vol. 3: Cell Mediated Reactions. Miscellaneous Topics.
VIII + 160 p., 7 fig., 12 tab., 1982. ISBN 3-8055-0960-X

National Library of Medicine, Cataloging in Publication
Idiopathic, food-induced, and drug-induced pseudo-allergic reactions /
Editors, P. Dukor . . . [et al.]. – Basel; New York: Karger, 1985. –
(Pseudo-allergic reactions; v. 4)
Includes bibliographies and index.
1. Drug Hypersensitivity 2. Food Hypersensitivity 3. Hypersensitivity I. Dukor, P. (Peter) II. Series
W1 PS123M v. 4 [WD 300 I19]
ISBN 3-8055-3798-0

Drug Dosage

The authors and the publisher have exerted every effort to ensure that drug selection and dosage set forth in this text are in accord with current recommendations and practice at the time of publication. However, in view of ongoing research, changes in government regulations, and the constant flow of information relating to drug therapy and drug reactions, the reader is urged to check the package insert for each drug for any change in indications and dosage and for added warnings and precautions. This is particularly important when the recommended agent is a new and/or infrequently employed drug.

Printed in Switzerland by Werner Druck AG, Basel
ISBN 3-8055-3798-0

Contents

Allergomimetic Reactions to Food and Pseudo-Food-Allergy

Hyperventilation and Pseudo-Allergic Reactions

Malignant Hyperpyrexia

Immunologic Abnormalities Induced by *D*-Penicillamine

Acknowledgement

Dr. *Peter Dukor* is, due to increasing other commitments, not able to continue his work as co-editor of the PAR-series. We would like to express our sincerest thanks for his friendship and stimulating cooperation.

P. Kallós
H.D. Schlumberger
G.B. West

PAR. Pseudo-Allergic Reactions. Involvement of Drugs and Chemicals, vol. 4, pp. 1–12 (Karger, Basel 1985)

Introduction

P. Kallós, H.D. Schlumberger, G.B. West

Helsingborg, Sweden; Wuppertal, FRG; Epsom, Surrey, Great Britain

The fourth volume of PAR documents the viability and acceptance of this new concept. Moreover, the reviews in the present volume show that pseudo-allergic reactions lie at the bottom of some disorders which hitherto were not recognized as allergomimetic states. For example, the first two reviews deal with 'Hereditary Angioedema' (*Laurell)* and 'Idiopathic and Exercise-Induced Anaphylaxis' (*Sonin and Patterson).*

Hereditary angioedema, an autosomal dominant trait, was described by *Osler* [50] as early as in 1888. Since then, tremendous progress has been achieved. This inherited pseudo-allergic disease is due to the deficiency or inactivity of a regulatory protein of the complement system, $C\bar{1}$-esterase inhibitor ($C\bar{1}$-INH). The biochemical events leading to the occurrence of 'spontaneous' attacks of angioedema, a type-I allergomimetic reaction, have been well defined and are exhaustively discussed by *Laurell* [see also 5, 20]. The unique feature of the variant forms of this disorder is that the continuous administration of testosterone derivatives with attenuated androgenic activity, such as danazol, normalizes $C\bar{1}$-INH production in the majority of cases, thus preventing attacks. In a few cases (about 2%) of hereditary angioedema (as in some other hereditary complement-component deficiencies), signs and symptoms of lupus erythematosus occur [55]. In such a case, danazol-treatment has been able to reverse both syndromes [45].

The second group of disorders, denoted 'idiopathic anaphylaxis', is according to *Sonin and Patterson* undoubtedly of pseudo-allergic nature. In contrast to hereditary angioedema, neither the genetic nor the molecular mechanisms of these disorders are known. There is symptomatic therapy only. It is definitely established, however, that the reactions which can lead to life-threatening (rarely fatal) respiratory and circulatory shock are *not* IgE-mediated allergic processes. 'Anaphylaxis' is thus a misnomer, but generally used in the literature. It is to be hoped that the review by *Sonin and Patterson* will lead to increased recognition of these syndromes and to further investigations of their pathomechanism. As *Sonin and Patterson* stress, a number of cases suffer from food-dependent exercise anaphylaxis. The pseudo-allergic syndrome occurs in connection with postprandial exercise. Patients and their doctors tend to ascribe the disorder to food allergy, an area reviewed in the present volume by *Pearson and Rix.* These authors point out that food allergy was from the beginning a somewhat ill-defined concept. Signs and symptoms observed after a meal were often regarded by patients and their physicians as due to a specific food. Moreover, without investigations into the pathomechanism or on the basis of overestimated 'positive' prick- or intracutaneous tests with food extracts, an allergic origin of the disorders was postulated, regardless of the nature of symptoms. The early history of these erratic and dangerous tendencies is reviewed by *Pearson and Rix.*

The fact that ingested food is able to elicit an allergic disorder, characterized by urticaria, conjunctivitis, rhinitis, asthma and vomiting, was proven beyond doubt in the classical investigations by *Prausnitz and Küstner* [52] described in 1921. They showed that the intracutaneous injection of an extract of the eliciting food, muscle of bony fish, caused in the allergic subject an immediate local wheal and erythema, and this did not occur in controls. Moreover, an intracutaneous injection of 0.1 ml serum of the fish-allergic subject was able to 'sensitize' the skin of naive individuals. The skin site so prepared reacted 24 h later with wheal and erythema to fish extract injected into it. The specificity of this passively transferred allergic reactivity has been convincingly documented by the authors. The nature of the transferred 'principle' was not clarified at that time. The authors showed, however, that it was not a complement-fixing or precipitating antibody. As is well known, it was later shown to be a certain class of immunoglobulins, IgE.

Despite the description of this well-documented case of food allergy and a most reliable diagnostic method, an abundance of papers has been published in this area, again based on anamnesis, clinical observations, open elimination-diets, re-introduction diets, and overestimated skin tests with food extracts. Not only the syndrome observed by *Prausnitz and Küstner* [52] but also headache, migraine, fatigue, changes in mood and behavior, myalgia, arthralgia and rheumatoid arthritis were regarded as due to food allergy. A monograph, entitled 'Food Allergy', published in 1951 by *Rinkel, Randolph and Zeller* [53] provided a quasi-scientific basis for these claims for many years to come. This has been recently revived by one of the authors (*Randolph*) under the heading 'Clinical Ecology' [see *Pearson and Rix*]. It is perhaps of interest to note that one of us [37] published in the same year (1951) a detailed critical 'Editorial' on the monograph by *Rinkel* et al. [53], analyzing the theoretical basis of their statements, as a result of which the conclusions of *Rinkel* et al. [53] were unacceptable. According to *Rinkel* et al. [53], 'Food allergy in this monograph may be defined as a term used in reference to those foods for which it is possible to demonstrate a cause and effect relationship between the ingestion of a specific food and the production or accentuation of allergic symptoms. Thus, one is considered allergic to a food if it (a) produces headache; (b) increases hay fever; (c) induces asthma, or (d) gives rise to any other constant symptom pattern, providing these exhibit specificity.' *Kallós* [37] stressed that an *allergic* reaction cannot be characterized by the fact that a 'specific food' is supposed to elicit it, for example, in the form of headache. The allergic nature of a reaction is determined by the underlying mechanism; it is either mediated by specific antibodies or by specifically committed effector T lymphocytes. Moreover, it has been pointed out that *Rinkel* et al. [53] found by elimination-diet or open food-testing that about 20% of the population was allergic to cereals (such as wheat, rye) and that the signs and symptoms of hay-fever patients, allergic to rye pollen, were often aggravated during the pollen season by ingestion of rye bread or other cereal products. *Kallós* [37] described the results achieved by investigations on two groups of patients. Patients with hay fever, positive prick and provocation test to rye pollen, who claimed that rye bread aggravated their symptoms and also caused indigestion (nausea, vomiting, abdominal pain and/or diarrhoea) constituted one group; bakers with occupational allergic respiratory disease (rhinitis and/or asthma) due to inhalation of wheat flour and/or rye flour, with positive prick and provocation test, who also claimed that the ingestion of cereal products elicited symptoms of their respiratory disorder and indigestion, fatigue and headache, constituted the other. In both groups, open food provocation elicited the signs and symptoms which the patients experienced before. Blind provocation with wheat flour, rye flour or bread, however, failed in all cases to provoke any pathological reaction. The patients were then convinced that they can eat cereal products with impunity and did so without exception [see also 9]. These results demonstrated the importance of the imagination of patients for the occurrence of symptoms, which were regarded then as due to a 'specific food'. Unfortunately, neither the 'Editorial', nor many other critical investigations could stop the 'food allergy fad'. The role of the permeability of the gut and that of 'mucosal immunity' for the prevention and elicitation of food allergy, were also neglected [for review see 22, 27, 34, 44, 58].

Pearson and Rix in the present volume analyze carefully the symptomatology of food allergy and define the diagnostic procedures which must be employed in an attempt to clarify cases with suspected food allergy. The elimination of suspected foods, often recommended by food faddists, can lead to dangerous qualitative and quantitative undernourishment. *Pearson and Rix* define the circumstances which lead to the fact that some food elicits in some individuals pseudo-allergic reactions, i.e. disorders, the symptoms of which mimic those of an allergic disease of any type, without being mediated by specific antibodies or cells (PAR to food). As they stress in their review, there are many patients, as well as their doctors, who claim that a specific food elicits symptoms in them, which are not allergomimetic but are nevertheless regarded as due to food allergy. These symptoms are often due to habitual hyperventilation leading to hypocarbia. By way of contrast *Pearson and Rix* denote this group as suffering from 'pseudo-food-allergy'. *Lum* has done pioneer research work on hyperventilation and the clinics of hypocarbia and his review in the present volume is therefore a most important contribution to the understanding, prevention and treatment of the numerous cases of pseudo-food-allergy. This apparently important and common syndrome was only cursorily mentioned in one recently published multi-authored report on food allergy [26] and not at all in another [27].

In a recent 'State of the Art' review [41], it has been stated that 'most medications can cause fever, with or without concomitant clinical manifestations'. Several different mechanisms for this effect were briefly mentioned, but it was concluded that 'the most common mechanism is probably an immunological reaction mediated by drug-induced antibodies'. Drug fever is a complex and puzzling disturbance of the homeostatic state and the above-mentioned immunologic mechanism is, in our opinion, uncommon. The maintenance of a constant body temperature (core temperature) of about 37 °C, is an important homeostatic function, which is effective at widely varying ambient temperature and humidity. Normally, exaggerated heat production, e.g. vigorous exercise, does not elevate body temperature to any great extent. Heat is a by-product of all metabolic processes. Even at rest striated musculature and other organs such as the liver produce most of the heat that is necessary for the maintenance of constant body temperature. On the other hand, heat is constantly lost through the body surface (mainly the skin) by radiation or convection and, predominantly, by evaporation of sweat. Thus, normal core temperature is maintained through a delicate balance between heat production and heat loss. This balance is governed by a nucleus in the preoptic region of the anterior hypothalamus which acts as a thermoregulatory center (TC). Excessive heat production leads via TC to peripheral vasodilatation and increased perspiration. In contrast, low ambient temperatures lead to vasoconstriction and diminished sweat production, eventually also to enhanced muscular activity, i.e. increased tone and/or shivering. The TC exerts its function through both the autonomic and somatic nervous systems [10, 23, 24, 42, 54, 56]. This thermoregulatory function implies the existence of some kind of a 'set point process' [10]. Elevated core temperature (fever between 37 and 41 °C) is a common symptom of bacterial and viral infections and inflammatory processes. Fever is not a result of a failure of the thermoregulatory mechanism. It occurs and is maintained for a time when a pyrogenic stimulus alters the TC and causes an upward shift of its set point. It was shown by *Beeson* [6] and *Bennet and Beeson* [7] as early as 1948 that pyrogenic stimuli, e.g. gram-negative bacteria and their endotoxin, do not act directly on the TC. Such exogenous pyrogens stimulate phagocytic cells, mainly circulating and sessile mononuclear phagocytes (i.e. Kupffer cells and splenic macrophages) to synthesize and release a polypeptide, denoted endogenous pyrogen (EP), which is the mediator of fever [2, 6, 7, 14, 19, 23, 24, 42, 54]. Fever research has been tremendously advanced by the isolation of the endotoxic and pyrogenic lipopolysacharide from the cell wall of Gram-negative bacteria by *Westphal and Lüderitz* [61] in 1953 and by its purification [60]. The lipid moiety, lipid A, stimulates the production of EP in vitro from phagocytic cells and in vivo, when injected intravenously. Fever occurs about 1 h after intravenous injection of lipid A [60]. Intravenous or intracarotid injection of EP induces a 'brisk fever' after a much shorter latent period of 5–10 min [19]. EP is a polypeptide of 11,000 molecular weight, which has recently been purified to homogeneity [40]. It is identical with the monokine lymphocyte-activating factor which is able to potentiate the response of T lymphocytes to mitogens. This factor was originally described by *Gery and Waksman* [28] in 1972. It is now denoted Interleukin 1 (IL 1) [19, 21, 40, 57]. This means that EP is involved in important immuno-regulatory processes and that fever can be regarded as a defence mechanism which facilitates the production of acute phase proteins [29, 51] and the clonal expansion of antigen-stimulated T lymphocytes, which then secrete Interleukin 2 (lymphocyte growth factor). Thus, very old concepts regarding the beneficial effects of fever must be revived and re-investigated [for references see 19, 21, 40, 60, 63].

EP shifts the set point of the TC upwards by locally stimulating the cyclooxygenase pathway of arachidonic acid metabolism, leading to the production of pyrogenic prostaglandin E_2. This also explains that cyclo-oxygenase inhibitors, such as the majority of non-steroidal anti-inflammatory drugs (NSAIDs) including acetylsalicylic acid (ASA), are effective in preventing or terminating fever. They do not influence the production of EP, but its effect. According to recent results of *Baracos* et al. [4], EP stimulates the production of prostaglandin E_2 in skeletal muscles. PgE_2 enhances considerably intralysosomal proteolysis in the muscle. These processes lie at the bottom of the negative nitrogen balance and myalgia, often observed in febrile subjects, and these are also inhibited by NSAIDs [4]. Monoamines, cyclic AMP and ionic interchanges also probably play roles in the action of EP on TC [19, 23, 24, 42, 54].

The circumstances under which allergic mechanisms lead to EP production and fever have been defined by *Bernheim* et al. [8]. Circulating immune complexes of suitable size, consisting of antigen, antibody (IgG) with or without complement, stimulate mononuclear phagocytes to EP production and elicit fever. This mechanism is operating, for example, in serum sickness [8] and in a few cases of penicillin allergy [12]. IgE is not able to mediate febrile reactions. Antigen-stimulated T cells secrete soluble factors (lymphokines) some of which stimulate EP synthesis and release. An example is tuberculin-fever in tuberculous or BCG-vaccinated humans and animals [8]. It is certain that antibody-mediated allergic drug fever is uncommon.

Drugs can have pyrogenic properties and cause fever in susceptible hosts without engaging allergic mechanisms. The anti-tumor agent, bleomycin, was shown to elicit fever in about 25% of treated patients, often a few hours after the first administration. In patients with lymphoma, the frequency was much higher, up to 90%. The affected patients experienced chills, shivering, hypotension, respiratory distress and fever (39–41 °C), a state resembling endotoxin or anaphylactoid shock. *Dinarello* et al. [18, 19] showed that bleomycin is able to stimulate phagocytes of rabbits and susceptible humans to synthesize and release EP, thereby eliciting fever.

Other drugs and chemicals exert pyrogenic activitiy in a similar way. A corticosteroid derivative, 5-β-hydrogen-etiocholanolone, elicits EP-fever in humans, but in no other species. The corresponding 5-α-derivative is inactive. An immuno-stimulating (adjuvant) compound, muramyl-dipeptide, and the interferon inducer, polyinosinic-polycytodylic acid, are highly pyrogenic for humans and animals by stimulating EP synthesis and release [for references see 19]. Drug fever has been observed as an occupational disease in a number of workers in a pharmaceutical plant producing streptokinase. The workers inhaled dust of the drug and about 25% of them reacted after 2–3 h at work with chills and fever due to EP [38]. Direct stimulation of EP synthesis and release is probably the mechanism which lies at the bottom of most cases of drug fever, in which the thermoregulatory processes remain intact, but the set point of TC is shifted upwards. The results briefly described here make the importance of the genetic make-up of the reacting organism apparent. It should be stressed once again that even when shock-like symptoms occur, no allergic mechanisms are involved in the elicitation of drug fever.

In another group of cases, pharmacogenetic fever is due to a failure of the thermoregulatory mechanism, EP and TC being most probably not involved, at least primarily. Body temperature in such cases is often extremely elevated and lies between 41 and 46 °C. A fatal outcome is not uncommon and antipyretic NSAIDs are without effect [for references see 10, 11, 19, 42, 56]. This kind of extreme temperature elevation is denoted hyperpyrexia (or hyperthermia), in some instances with the prefix 'malignant'.

Malignant hyperpyrexia (MH), as it occurs in susceptible subjects (MHS) in response to general anaesthesia, is reviewed in the present volume by *Halsall and Ellis.* The main eliciting drugs are the depolarizing muscle-relaxant, suxamethonium, and the volatile anaesthetic, halothane. MH occurred in some cases after the administration of suxamethonium alone, but in the majority of cases both drugs were given.

Suxamethonium is a histamine releaser and therapeutic doses elicit pseudo-allergic (anaphylactoid) reactions in susceptible individuals [1, 25, 33, 39, 64]. This property of the drug has no relevance to its MH-eliciting effect.

Susceptibility to MH is an autosomal dominant hereditary trait, its phenotypical expression being, according to *Halsall and Ellis,* an often subclinical myopathy originally described by *Denborough* et al. [16] in 1970. This myopathy deeply influences the excitability and metabolism of skeletal muscles. Under the influence of the eliciting drugs, sudden contraction, rigidity and excessive heat production occur, leading to rapid elevation of the core temperature. EP and TC are not involved. The clinical signs and symptoms and the pathophysiological processes involved in MH are described by *Halsall and Ellis.* Despite intense research, there is no consensus concerning the pathomechanism of the syndrome, the outcome of which is still fatal in about 30% of cases. Hyperpyrexia is the result of an 'acute catabolic crisis' [11]. This is manifested in the musculature by a sudden and considerable rise in the concentration of Ca^{2+} in the myoplasm. Knowledge of this early event has made it possible to successfully use drugs which lower myoplasmic calcium levels, such as dantrolene-sodium, in the treatment of MH. Other such drugs, e.g. procaine and verapamil, are less effective [11, 48]. Drugs which elevate myoplasmic calcium levels, such as cardiac glycosides and caffeine, worsen the syndrome. Antipyretic NSAIDs are ineffective. Intense physical cooling is an important adjunct in the treatment. As *Halsall and Ellis* point out, it is of great importance to identify MHS subjects. Biopsied muscle samples contract in vitro under the influence of 3% halothane, which does not contract muscle of non-susceptible individuals. This important diagnostic method was introduced by *Ellis* and his co-workers. Research in this area has also been promoted by the discovery that certain breeds of swine are also susceptible to MH. The syndrome occurs in them under the influence of suxamethonium and/or halothane, but also, as *Halsall and Ellis* point out, under stressful conditions [see also 47, 49]. Excised striated muscle of MHS swine contracts under the influence of halothane. MH in stressful situations has been observed in many other animal species [47], and extreme stress is perhaps also an elicitor of MH in susceptible humans [62].

Denborough et al. [17] recently investigated muscle biopsy specimens of 15 parents of 13 infants who died in the 'sudden infant death syndrome' (cot death). Five muscle samples showed a contraction when exposed to 3% halothane, a reaction characteristic for MHS. The connection between the two syndromes is, however, as pointed out by *Halsall and Ellis,* still uncertain. At least some cases of cot death are, according to *Coombs and McLaughlan* [13], due to anaphylaxis, induced in infants allergic to cow's milk by regurgitation and aspiration of milk proteins. The 'enigma of cot death' [13] is very complex. According to *Halsall and Ellis* the post mortem core temperature of cot death babies is often higher than expected and 'changes in small blood vessels consistent with heat stroke have been described'. Heat stroke is due to the failure of heat loss at extreme ambient temperature and humidity [56], in contrast to MH, where extreme heat production causes the hyperpyrexia. Despite this difference, it has recently been found that intravenous dantrolene-sodium is an effective remedy in cases of heat stroke [15, 43].

Neuroleptic drugs, such as phenothiazines, butyrophenones and thioxanthenes, are also able to induce extreme, sometimes fatal, hyperpyrexia, which is possibly due to damage to and dysfunction of TC, leading to thermoregulatory failure [3, 30, 31, 35, 36, 59].

Allergic mechanisms are thus not involved in the elicitation of MH.

The last review in this volume, by *Smith and Hammarström,* deals with the effect of *D*-penicillamine on the immune system. Penicillamine, originally introduced in the therapy of Wilson's disease as a chelating agent, is now mainly used as an anti-inflammatory drug in the treatment of rheumatoid arthritis. As *Huskisson* [36] stressed in his review of the pharmacology of penicillamine, this drug has, in contrast to other NSAIDs and corticosteroids, a specific effect on the course of rheumatoid arthritis, which is achieved after some months of administration. Also in contrast to corticosteroids and ASA-like NSAIDs, penicillamine does not interfere with arachidonic acid metabolism. In rare cases, penicillamine induces the production of antibodies against acetylcholine receptors and thereby the signs and symptoms of myasthenia gravis. This adverse effect of penicillamine was briefly discussed in volume 3 of this series [46]. Many new facts have been uncovered since then [32] and an exhaustive review of the effects of penicillamine on the immune system was warranted. Important differences between the idiopathic and the penicillamine-induced myasthenia syndrome have been detected. Most interesting is perhaps the difference in HLA associations. According to *Smith and Hammarström,* in idiopathic cases, a significantly increased frequency of the HLA B8/Dw3/DR3 antigens has been found, whereas penicillamine-induced cases showed a prevalence of Bw35/DR1. Penicillamine also induces a number of other autoallergic disorders, which are thoroughly reviewed by *Smith and Hammarström.* A main feature of all these disorders is that no immune activity is directed against penicillamine itself. Therefore, the autoallergic disorders thus induced are not due to 'penicillamine allergy' and must be regarded as pseudo-allergic processes.

We are aware that more problems are posed than solved in the areas dealt with in the present volume. Hopefully, the PAR concept can add to the understanding of the still controversial pathomechanism of some of the disorders discussed and stimulate further research.

References

1 Assem, E.S.K.; Frost, P.G.; Levis, R.D.: Anaphylactic-like reactions to suxamethonium. Anaesthesia *36:* 405–410 (1981).

2 Atkins, E.; Bodel, P.; Francis, L.: Release of endogenouos pyrogen in vitro from rabbit mononuclear cells. J. exp. Med. *126:* 357–383 (1967).

3 Ayd, F.J.: Fatal hyperpyrexia during chlorpromazine therapy. J. clin. exp. Psychopath. *17:* 189–192 (1956).

4 Barracos, V.; Rodemann, P.; Dinarello, C.A.; Goldberg, A.L.: Stimulation of muscle protein degradation and prostaglandin E_2 release – by leucocytic pyrogen (Interleukin 1). New Engl. J. Med. *308:* 553–558 (1983).

5 Becker, E.L.: Nature and classification of immediate-type allergic reactions. Adv. Immunol. *13:* 267–313 (1971).

6 Beeson, P.B.: Temperature elevating effect of a substance obtained from polymorphonuclear leucocytes. J. clin. Invest. *27:* 524 (1948).

7 Bennet, L.L., Jr.; Beeson, P.B.: Studies on the pathogenesis of fever. Parts I and II. J. exp. Med. *98:* 477–508 (1953).

8 Bernheim, H.A.; Francis, L.; Atkins, E.: Hypersensitivity fever: cell-mediated and antibody-mediated mechanisms; in Lipton, Fever, pp. 11–21 (Raven Press, New York 1980).

9 Blands, J.; Diamant, B.; Kallós, P.; Kallós-Deffner, L.; Löwenstein, H.: Flour allergy in bakers. Int. Archs Allergy appl. Immun. *52:* 392–406 (1975).

10 Bligh, J.: Central neurology of homeothermy and fever; in Lipton, Fever, pp. 81–89 (Raven Press, New York 1980).

11 Britt, B.A.: Etiology and pathophysiology of malignant hyperthermia. Fed. Proc. *38:* 44–48 (1979).

12 Chusid, M.J.; Atkins, E.: Studies on the mechanism of penicillin-induced fever. J. exp. Med. *136:* 227–240 (1972).

13 Coombs, R.R.A.; McLaughlan, P.: The enigma of cot death: is the modified anaphylaxis hypothesis an explanation for some cases? Lancet *i:* 1388–1389 (1982).

14 Cranston, W.I.; Goodale, F.; Snell, E.S.; Wendt, F.: The role of leucocytes in the initial action of bacterial pyrogens in man. Clin. Sci. *15:* 219–225 (1956).

15 Denborough, M.A.: Heat stroke and malignant hyperpyrexia. Med. J. Aust. *i:* 204–205 (1982).

16 Denborough, M.A.; Ebeling, P.; King, J.O.; Zapf, P.: Myopathy and malignant hyperpyrexia. Lancet *i:* 1138–1140 (1970).

17 Denborough, M.A.; Galloway, G.J.; Hopkinson, K.C.: Malignat hyperpyrexia and sudden infant death. Lancet *ii:* 1068–1069 (1982).

18 Dinarello, C.A.; Ward, S.B.; Wolff, S.M.: Pyrogenic properties of bleomycin. Cancer Chemother. Rep. *57:* 393–398 (1973).

19 Dinarello, C.A.; Wolff, S.M.: Molecular basis of fever in humans. Am. J. Med. *72:* 799–819 (1982).

20 Donaldson, V.H.; Evans, R.R.: A biochemical abnormality in hereditary angioedema: absence of serum inhibitor of C1 esterase. Am. J. Med. *35:* 37–44 (1963).

21 Duff, G.W.; Durum, S.K.: The pyrogenic and mitogenic actions of Interleukin 1 are related. Nature, Lond. *304:* 449–451 (1983).

22 Enerbäck, L.: The gut mucosal mast cell. Monogr. Allergy, vol. 17, pp. 222–232 (Karger, Basel 1981).

23 Feldberg, W.S.; Milton, A.S.: Prostaglandins and body temperature. Handbook of experimental pharmacology, vol. 50 I, pp 617–656 (Springer, Heidelberg 1978).

24 Ferreira, S.H.; Vane, J.R.: Mode of action of antiinflammatory drugs which are prostaglandin-synthetase inhibitors. Handbook of experimental pharmacology, vol. 50 II, pp. 348–398 (Springer, Heidelberg 1979).

25 Fisher, M.M.; More, D.G.: The epidemiology and clinical features of anaphylactic reactions in anaesthesia. Anaesth. intensive Care *9:* 226–234 (1981).

26 Food intolerance and food aversion. A joint report of the Royal College of Physicians and the British Nutrition Foundation. J. R. Coll. Physns, Lond. *18:* 83–123 (1984).

27 Food sensitivity. Proceedings of a 'Marabou Symposium', Sundbyberg 1983. Nutr. Rev. *42:* 65–140 (1984).

28 Gery, I.; Waksman, B.H.: Potentiation of T-lymphocyte response to mitogens: the cellular source of potentiating mediators. J. exp. Med. *136:* 143–152 (1972).

29 Gewurz, H.: The biology of C-reactive protein; in Dixon, Fisher, The biology of immunologic disease, pp. 139–154 (HP, New York 1983).

30 Giller, G.; Greydanus, D.E.: Haloperidol induced comatose state with hyperthermia and rigidity in adolescents: two case reports with a literature-review. J. clin. Psychiat. *40:* 102–103 (1979).

31 Greenblatt, B.J.; Rogers-Greenblatt, G.: Chlorpromazine and hyperthermia. Clin. Pediat. *12:* 504–505 (1973).

32 Grob, B. (ed.): Myasthenia gravis. Ann. N.Y. Acad. Sci. *377* (1981).

33 Grob, D.; Lilienthal, J.L.; Harvey, A.M.: On certain vascular effects of curare in man. The 'histamine reaction'. Bull. Johns Hopkins Hosp. *80:* 299–322 (1947).

34 Hanson, L.Å.: Mucosal immunity. Ann. N.Y. Acad. Sci. *409:* 1–21 (1983).

35 Hunziker, T.; Fehlmann, U.; Kummer, H.; Spengler, H.; Hoigné, R.: Arzneifieber auf das Antidepressivum Nomifensin (Alival). Schweiz. med. Wschr. *110:* 1295–1300 (1980).

36 Huskisson, E.C.: Penicillamine and drugs with a specific action in rheumatoid arthritis. Handbook of experimental Pharmacology, vol. 50 II, pp. 399–414 (Springer, Heidelberg 1979).

37 Kallós, P.: Nahrungsmittelallergie (food allergy). Editorial. Int. Archs Allergy appl. Immun. *2:* 76–82 (1951).

38 Kallós, P.: Introduction. Prog. Allergy, vol. 8, pp. VI–XVI (Karger, Basel 1964).

39 Kallós, P.; Kallós, L.: Histamine and some other mediators of pseudoallergic reactions. PAR. Pseudo-allergic reactions. Involvement of drugs and chemicals, vol. 1, pp. 28–55 (Karger, Basel 1980).

40 Lachman, L.B.; Maizel, A.L.: Human immunoregulatory molecules: Interleukin 1, Interleukin 2 and B-cell growth factor. Contemp. Top. mol. Immunol. *9:* 147–167 (1983).

41 Lipsky, B.A.; Hirschman, J.V.: Drug fever (state of the art review). J. Am. med. Ass. *245:* 851–854 (1981).

42 Lomax, P.; Schönbaum, E.; Jacob, J. (eds.): Temperature regulation and drug action (Karger, Basel 1975).

43 Lydiatt, G.S.; Hill, G.E.: Treatment of heat stroke with dantrolene. J. Am. med. Ass. *246:* 41–42 (1981).

44 McGhee, J.R.; Mestecky, J. (eds.): The secretory immune system. Ann. N.Y. Acad. Sci. *409:* (1983).
45 Masse, R.; Younion, P.; Dorval, J.C.; Cledes, J.: Reversal of lupus erythematosus-like disease with danazol. Lancet *ii:* 651 (1980).
46 Mastaglia, F.L.; Argov, Z.: Immunologically mediated drug-induced neuromuscular diseases. PAR. Pseudo-allergic reactions. Involvement of drugs and chemicals, vol. 3, pp. 62–86 (Karger, Basel 1982).
47 Mitchell, G.; Heffron, L.L.A.: Porcine stress syndromes. Adv. Food Res. *28:* 167–230 (1982).
48 Moulds, K.F.W.; Denborough, M.A.: Procaine in malignant hyperpyrexia. Br. med. J. *i:* 526–528 (1972).
49 Okumura, P.; Crocker, B.D.; Denborough, M.A.: Identification of susceptibility to malignant hyperpyrexia in swine. Br. J. Anaesth. *51:* 171–176 (1979).
50 Osler, W.: Hereditary angio-neurotic edema. Am. J. med. Sci. *95:* 362–367 (1888).
51 Pepys, M.B.: C-reactive protein fifty years on. Lancet *i:* 663–667 (1981).
52 Prausnitz, C.; Küstner, H.: Studien über die Überempfindlichkeit. Zentbl. Bakt. I. Orig. *86:* 160–169 (1921).
53 Rinkel, H.J.; Randolph, T.G.; Zeller, M.: Food allergy (Thomas, Springfield 1951).
54 Rosendorff, B.; Woolf, J.: Inhibition of fever. Hand. exp. Pharmac., vol. 50, part II, pp. 255–279 (Springer, Heidelberg 1979).
55 Rother, U.; Till, G.; Voigtländer, V.; Hänsch, G.: The complement system. PAR. Pseudo-allergic reactions. Involvement of drugs and chemicals, vol. 2, pp. 71–104 (Karger, Basel 1980).
56 Simon, H.B.: Extreme pyrexia in man; Lipton, Fever, pp. 213–224 (Raven Press, New York 1980).
57 Simon, P.L.; Willoughby, W.F.: Biochemical and biological characterization of rabbit Interleukin 1. Lymphokines *6:* 47–60 (1982).
58 Stober, W.; Hanson, L.Å.; Sell, K.W. (eds.): Recent advances in mucosal immunity (Raven Press, New York 1982).
59 Westlake, R.J.; Rastegar, A.: Hyperpyrexia from drug combinations. J. Am. med. Ass. *225:* 1250 (1973).
60 Westphal, O.; Jann, K.; Himmelspach, K.: Chemistry and immunochemistry of bacterial lipopolysaccharides as cell-wall antigens and endotoxins. Prog. Allergy, vol. 33, pp. 9–39 (Karger, Basel 1983).
61 Westphal, O.; Lüderitz, O.: Chemische Erforschung von Lipopolysacchariden gramnegativer Bakterien. Angew. Chem. *66:* 407–417 (1953)
62 Wingard, D.W.: Malignant hyperthermia: a common stress syndrome? Lancet *ii:* 1450–1451 (1974).
63 Wolstenholme, G.E.W.; Birch, J. (eds.): Pyrogens and fever (Churchill, Edinburgh 1971).
64 Youngman, P.R.; Taylor, K.M.; Wilson, J.D.: Anaphylactoid reactions to neuromuscular blocking agents. Lancet *ii:* 597–599 (1983).

Paul Kallós, MD, Villatomtsvägen 12, S-252 34 Helsingborg (Sweden)
H.D. Schlumberger, MD, Institut für Immunologie und Onkologie, Bayer AG, Friedrich-Ebert-Strasse 217, D-5600 Wuppertal 1 (FRG)
G.B. West, MD, 22 Burgh Heath Road, GB-Epsom, Surrey KT17 4LS (England)

PAR. Pseudo-Allergic Reactions. Involvement of Drugs and Chemicals, vol. 4, pp. 13–46 (Karger, Basel 1985)

C$\bar{1}$-Inhibitor Dysfunction and Complement Activation in Hereditary and Acquired Angioedema

Anna-Brita Laurell

Department of Medical Microbiology, Lund, Sweden

Introduction

Distinct from angioedema due to type-I allergic reaction, there exist variant forms of the disease not mediated by IgE, and where other mechanisms must account for the symptoms. Of this category, hereditary angioedema (HAE) is a well-defined syndrome, clearly representing a pseudo-allergic reaction (PAR) [8, 50, 79], due to an inborn deficiency of one of the regulatory proteins within the complement system, the C$\bar{1}$-inhibitor (C$\bar{1}$-INH).

In a miscellaneous group of angioedema patients, with or without symptoms of urticaria, that cannot be categorized as having a type-I allergic reaction, there are also those in whom an acquired C$\bar{1}$-INH deficiency has been demonstrated. It is not clear whether all such cases should be regarded as PARs, as disorders within the immune system may also be present in some of them. In this survey of HAE, and angioedema with acquired C$\bar{1}$-INH deficiency, attention will also be focused on reported cases of other disorders within the complement system, where angioedema has been a more or less pronounced feature.

The Complement System (C System)

Complement is a complex system of normal plasma proteins that, when activated, give rise to a cascade reaction similar to that of the blood coagulation process. The system is composed of 20 distinct plasma proteins, six of which are regulating plasma proteins responsible for checking distinct steps in the sequential reactions. Details of the factors of the C system and of their activation and control mechanisms are available in comprehensive surveys [53, 81, 88, 110, 122, 148].

In the brief survey which follows, attention has been focussed on the activation of the classical pathway and the steps involved (fig. 1), since an understanding of these is central to attempts at clarifying the pathogenesis of HAE, and certain types of acquired angioedema.

The first C factor, C1, is a macromolecular Ca^{2+}-dependent complex of three protein subcomponents, C1q, C1r and C1s [107, 121].C1q in the complex binds to the Fc part of IgM and IgG antibodies in immune complexes [121], which results in the activation to enzymes of, first, C1r and then C1s, both of which belong to the serine esterases [106, 143, 176]. Activated C1 and C1s are known as C1 esterase. In addition to immune complexes, other activators – such as certain viruses, bacteria, carbohydrates and endotoxins – are capable of transforming C1 to C1 esterase [11, 32, 33, 111, 158]. Complexes of C-reactive protein and certain polycations bind C1q and activate C1r and C1s [26, 80, 160, 161]. Enzymes, such as trypsin and plasmin, have been shown to activate C1 [141]. Active C1 esterase cleaves the next factor in the classical pathway, C4, into two fragments, C4a and C4b [19, 132]. The larger fragment, C4b, can bind to cells and to structures on IgG and IgM in immune complexes and, by means of another structure in the C4b molecule, it is also capable of binding the next factor in the complement sequence, C2, thus forming a C4bC2 complex. C2 is now cleaved by the activated $C\bar{1}s$ into two fragments, C2a and C2b [61, 138]. The resulting complex, C4b2a ($C\overline{42}$), has enzymatic activity and is the C3 convertase of the classical pathway. During the cleavage of C2, a fragment with kinin-like activity is released into the fluid phase [105].

C4b2a splits the next component, C3, into C3a and C3b [15, 123].C3a is a biologically highly active protein with a molecular weight of 9,000 that releases histamine from mast cells and basophilic leukocytes [15, 72]. The larger fragment, C3b, can bind to cells and immune complexes and together with C4b2a, a new enzyme, C5 convertase is formed that cleaves C5 into the C5a and C5b fragments [34, 128]. C5a is a peptide with a molecular weight of 17,000 [34]. It has chemotactic activity and acts as an anaphylatoxin, releasing histamine from mast cells and basophils [72]; it also causes aggregation of polymorphonuclear leukocytes [37, 40, 73]. C5b, the larger fragment, can bind to surface of cells and then the components C6, C7, C8 and C9 associate in an non-enzymatic manner with C5b

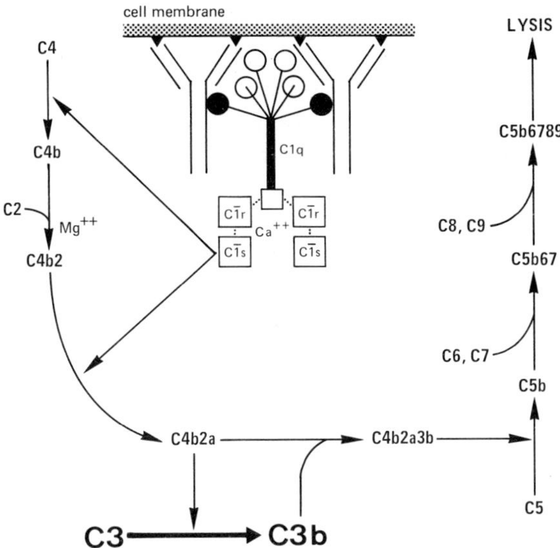

Fig. 1. Activation of the classical pathway. A bar over a factor indicates activation. [Reproduced with permission from Dr. *U. Johnson:* On different activation mechanisms of the human complement system; thesis Lund, 1981.]

resulting in a large complex, the membrane attack complex (MAC), C5b-C9 [137, 169]. When MAC is formed on the membranes of cells by binding of C5b, changes occur in the lipid bilayer of the membrane resulting in lysis of the cell [12, 85, 115, 137].

The C4b2a complex is labile because of the rapid decay of C2a [123]. The biological function of C4b is controlled by a normal plasma protein, factor I (C3b inactivator) [87, 149, 168], which in the presence of a cofactor, C4 binding protein (C4BP), splits C4b into C4c and C4d [31, 154].

The earlier steps of complement activation by the classical pathway are checked by the C1̄-INH [108, 140]. On activation of C1 by various activators (immune complexes, CRP complexes, enzymes), complexes of C1̄r-C1̄s-C1̄-INH are formed by binding of C1̄-INH to C1̄r-C1̄s and dissociation of the C1̄r-C1̄s-C1̄-INH complex from C1q [3, 22, 96, 100, 102, 179].

Since C$\bar{1}$s in the complex is unable to attack C4 and C2, the binding of C$\bar{1}$-INH to activated C1 thus controls the first step in the classical pathway. It has also been shown that C$\bar{1}$r-C$\bar{1}$s-C$\bar{1}$-INH is present in normal serum, indicating a continuous physiological activation of C1, which is regulated by the C$\bar{1}$-INH [99, 100, 175]. The foregoing may provide a clue to the understanding of the periodicity of symptoms in angioedema with C$\bar{1}$-INH deficiency and the factors known to cause them; this will be expanded on below.

C$\bar{1}$ Inhibitor

The C$\bar{1}$-INH was first described by *Ratnoff and Lepow* [140] and characterized further by *Levy and Lepow* [108] and by *Pensky* et al. [134]. A protein termed α_2-neuraminoglycoprotein, isolated by *Schultze* et al. [159], was later shown to be identical with C$\bar{1}$-INH [133]. C$\bar{1}$–INH is labile when heated to 60 °C, and is irreversibly inactivated at pH below 6. It has α_2-electrophoretic mobility. With a carbohydrate content of 35%, it is the most carbohydrate-rich glycoprotein present in serum [68]. The molecular weight is 10,500 [66, 67].

C$\bar{1}$-INH binds stoichiometrically to C1r and C1s, thereby inhibiting their enzymatic activity [22, 134, 176, 177].

The only known inhibitor of C$\bar{1}$r and C$\bar{1}$s is the C$\bar{1}$-INH, which has also been shown to inhibit activated Hageman factor, plasmin, kallikrein, and factor X1a (activated plasma thromboplastin antecedent) [54, 63, 78, 142].

C$\bar{1}$-INH is the major inhibitor of activated Hageman factor and kallikrein [54, 63]. Kallikrein is inhibited also by α_2-macroglobulin [65] and α_1-antitrypsin [56]. The main inhibitor of plasmin is α_2-antiplasmin [28, 124, 125]. Factor X1a is regulated by antithrombin III.

C$\bar{1}$-INH is synthesized by the hepatocytes [75], its plasma concentration being 17 mg/ml. The normal range is 72–153% of a normal standard pool [162].

Hereditary Angioedema

In a large family study, *Osler* [130] reported the disease in patients spread over 5 generations, thus emphasizing the hereditary nature of the disease. Patients with HAE suffer from recurrent attacks of circumscribed, non-itching edema in the skin, in the gastrointestinal tract (mimicking acute abdominal disorders), and in the respiratory tract where it results in laryngeal edema often with fatal outcome. The onset of the disease has been reported to occur from early childhood up to 50 or 60 years of age but is most frequent in adolescence – often in menarchal girls [46]. Reports of 3 large Swedish families show variations in the severity of attacks during pregnancy and puerperium [14]. The duration of attacks usually varies between 1 and 3 days, but may be longer.

Landerman et al. [90] found that a serum control factor of kallikrein was missing in HAE. In a classical paper, *Donaldson and Evans* [44] showed that in HAE patients $C\bar{1}$-INH was lacking in the blood, or only present in very low concentrations. They also showed that the disease is inherited as an autosomal dominant trait; thus those affected are heterozygous for the trait. Studies by *Johnson* et al. [75] showed that the low concentration of $C\bar{1}$-INH in HAE is the result of deficient synthesis in hepatic parenchymal cells, and that the disease was based on an inborn biosynthetic error.

As a consequence of the $C\bar{1}$-INH deficiency in HAE, the early steps of the classical pathway of complement activation are less well governed, which was clearly shown by *Donaldson and Evans* [44]. When C1 is activated, the serum concentrations of C4 and C2 decrease as a result of activation and secondary elimination from the fluid phase. C3, however, remains within the normal range [45], probably due to the ineffectiveness of the $C\overline{42}$ complex as a C3 convertase in free solution [123].

Trauma has been reported to cause the onset of HAE and of subsequent attacks, other causes being infections and even occasionally psychogenic factors [113]. Other precipitating events have also been discerned, such as hormonal factors, as attacks often occur in conjunction with menstrual periods [14, 46].

Mediators of Symptoms in HAE

Donaldson et al. [49] reported on a permeability-increasing activity in plasma obtained from HAE patients during attacks which could also be generated by incubating, at 37 °C, plasma obtained from the patients when they were free of symptoms. Intradermal injection of $C\bar{1}$s into healthy people produced swelling similar to that observed during HAE attacks [173]. From studies in which purified $C\bar{1}$s was injected into healthy people, or C2-deficient persons, and from experiments with C4-deficient guinea pigs, it was concluded that C4 and C2 were required for the kinin to be formed [82], and that the kinin, derived from C2, is clearly distinct from bradykinin [48, 83].

Injection of C$\bar{1}$s in individuals deficient in C4 or C2 failed to produce edema; in those with hereditary C3 deficiency, the edema response was the same as in healthy people [41]. Further evidence that the kinin in HAE is derived from C2 has recently been reported by *Bourgarit* et al. [16].

On the other hand, in an early study of HAE patients [90] decreased amounts of prekallikrein and signs of kallikrein activation were reported; kallikrein activation is caused by deficiency of C$\bar{1}$-INH, which is capable of blocking plasma kallikrein [142]. The broad inhibitor action of C$\bar{1}$-INH has been dealt with above. C$\bar{1}$-INH thus also interferes with activated Hageman factor (XIIa), factor X1a (plasma thromboplastin antecedent, PTA) and plasmin. That bradykinin was involved in the increased vascular permeability in HAE was suggested by *Talamo* et al. [167], who found increased amounts in plasma taken from patients during attacks. In recent studies it was postulated that activation of Hageman factor results in the activation of prekallikrein to kallikrein, and the release of bradykinin [153] which may cause the increased vascular permeability in HAE. *Schapira* et al. [152] found increased amounts of kallikrein antigen, complexed with plasma inhibitors that are able to block its action. *Curd* et al. [38] reported on the presence of kallikrein in induced blisters in HAE and on the generation of bradykinin by incubation of HAE plasma [39]. Against bradykinin as a possible mediator of the increased permeability, stands the fact that the edema in HAE is neither erythematous, itchy, nor painful.

The interaction between the complement and kallikrein systems, and the activation of Hageman factor and of plasmin, are intriguing problems in relation to the question of the mediator(s) in HAE. Activated Hageman factor can activate prekallikrein and plasminogen, and plasmin can activate C1 to C1 esterase [59]. On the other hand, neither C$\bar{1}$ nor activated C$\bar{1}$s are capable of activating Hageman factor or the plasmin or kallikrein systems. In addition to C$\bar{1}$, C$\bar{1}$-INH also inactivates the Hageman factor, plasmin and kallikrein, but it must be borne in mind that, as mentioned above, other important inhibitors of these enzymes also exist in plasma, while C$\bar{1}$-INH is the only known natural inhibitor of C$\bar{1}$. The interactions between the Hageman factor, the kallikrein and complement systems in plasma and the regulatory effect of C$\bar{1}$-INH are shown in figure 2.

Depending on the cause of an HAE attack, it may be reasonable to assume that the action of any of a variety of mediators may result in

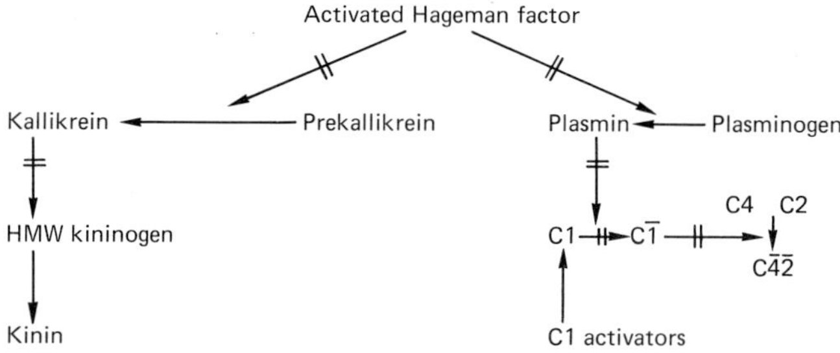

Fig. 2. Regulation by C1̄-INH of activation of the kallikrein, plasmin and complement systems. (Cross bars indicate inhibition by C1̄-INH.)

increased permeability in a given patient, as pointed out by *Donaldson* [43].

Genetic Variants of HAE

HAE is inherited as an autosomal dominant trait [44]. Most HAE patients either have low serum concentrations of C1̄-INH (< 30% of normal value, measured both with immunochemical and functional assays), but patients from several families have been described as having markedly increased concentrations in immunochemical tests. In these cases the C1̄-INH was found to be non-functioning, thus without effect in the esterolytic assay, and unable to inhibit the splitting of C4 by activated C1̄s [97, 101, 145, 146]. In another, more rare, group of patients, almost normal concentrations of non-functioning C1̄-INH were reported and, in the most rare form of the disease, a defective C1̄-INH protein that retains its inhibiting capacity in the esterolytic assay but fails to inhibit the action of activated C1 on C4 is synthesized in normal amounts [146].

In the most common form of HAE, type 1 (with low amounts of C1̄-INH in both assays), the protein has the same electrophoretic mobility as normal C1̄-INH (fig. 3). In all probability this is a reflection of the genetic background, those afflicted having one silent and one active gene. Whereas the C1̄-INH value in HAE patients during periods free from attacks might be assumed to be around 50% of normal, it is in fact 30% or less. The explanation for this may be as follows: In healthy people, the C1̄-INH concentration of 100% represents the amount remaining after about 30% of available C1̄-INH has already been consumed owing to complex formation with activated C1̄r-C1̄s, generated by constant physiological C1 activation

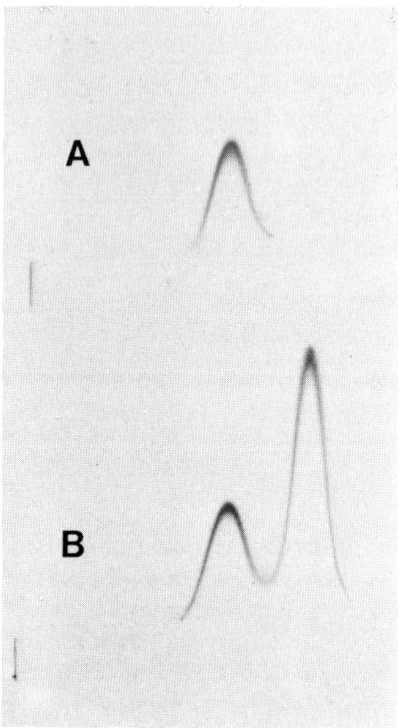

Fig. 3. Crossed immunoelectrophoresis of serum from a patient with HAE, variant form, type 2. The secondary electrophoretic step was run with anti-C$\bar{1}$-INH in the agarose gel. *A* Normal serum. *B* HAE serum.

[96, 102, 174, 175]. The magnitude of this physiological C1 activation is in all likelihood the same in HAE patients during symptom-free periods as in healthy people and thus, with an expected value corresponding to 60% of normal, the concentrations actually found would be around 30%.

Despite excessive activation of C1 during attacks, the amount of C$\bar{1}$r-C$\bar{1}$s-C$\bar{1}$-INH complexes is not markedly increased indicating that the reduced concentrations of C$\bar{1}$-INH available in these patients are probably completely consumed and do not suffice keeping the C1 activation under control. When the C$\bar{1}$-INH synthesis increases as a result of therapy (see below under 'Therapy'), the concentrations of C$\bar{1}$r-C$\bar{1}$s-C$\bar{1}$-INH increase correspondingly [99].

In the variant form of HAE, type 2, the content of non-functioning C$\bar{1}$-INH protein in plasma is very high, up to 200–400% of the normal. *Rosen* et al. [145] showed by immunoelectrophoresis that C$\bar{1}$-INH in sera from type-2 patients appeared in two molecular forms – one having the same electrophoretic mobility as normal C1̄-INH, and one with higher electrophoretic mobility. Using crossed immunoelectrophoresis, two distinct precipitation peaks were found (fig. 3) [4, 96]. The larger precipitation peak with α_1-electrophoretic mobility was found to be a complex between C1̄-INH protein and albumin [96], a finding also reported by *Rosen* et al. [146]. The reactivity of the abnormal C1̄-INH probably reflects a restrictive mutation of one of the C1̄-INH genes, resulting in the synthesis of C1̄-INH with a reactive SH group which interchanges with albumin. Analogous complex formations with albumin have been described for IgA molecules [170].

Concerning the two remaining types of HAE, with non-functioning C1̄-INH in normal or moderately decreased concentration and with normal electrophoretic mobility, nothing is known of the molecular changes resulting in the inactivity of the inhibitor. It is, however, reasonable to suppose that even here restrictive mutations have caused amino acid substitutions resulting in the synthesis of a non-functioning inhibitor.

Kallikrein is not inhibited by plasma from patients with conventional HAE, whereas significant kallikrein inhibition has been shown in some patients with the genetic variant form of HAE [63].

Association of HAE with Other Diseases

Lupus erythematosus-like disease as well as glomerulonephritis has been reported in increased frequency in HAE [47, 84]. It has been proposed that, owing to the chronic relative deficiency of C4 and C2 in HAE, the formation of C3 convertase is ineffective, thus predisposing to the development of immune complex disease – a predisposition analogous to that found in genetic deficiencies of C2 and C4 [89].

Laboratory Diagnosis of HAE

A diagnostic test procedure in the laboratory (table I) consists of immunochemical assays of C1̄-INH, C4 and C3 by Mancini assay or electroimmunoassay, analysis of C1̄-INH function using esterolytic tests [93, 94, 108], and analysis of the capacity of serum to inhibit C1̄s-mediated inactivation of C2 or C4 [62, 66]. *Ziccardi and Cooper* [180] have published a functional assay of C1̄-INH, based on the observation that C1̄-INH masks the antigenic properties of activated C1̄r [100, 178].

The characteristic C pattern in HAE is abnormal C1̄-INH in conjunction with low concentrations of C4 and C2; C1 activity is normal, as are the concentrations of C1 subcomponents and of C3.

Table I. Assays for diagnosis of HAE

Immunochemical
C1̄-INH, C1q, C3, C4: Electroimmunoassay [101, 102, 162]
Single radial immunodiffusion test [114]

Functional
C1̄-INH: Esterolytic test [93, 108]
Immunochemical functional assay [180]
Inhibition of C1̄s splitting activity on C4 [146]

In patients with recurrent attacks of angioedema, HAE should be suspected until excluded by laboratory diagnosis. As a rule, the procedure is simple and, in a preliminary screening, the immunochemical measurement of C1̄-INH and of C4 is discriminating: where both of these are within the normal range or increased, HAE may be excluded.

Further investigation will, however, be necessitated by any of the following three variations of the results of C1̄-INH, C4 and C3 analysis:

1. *Low value of C1̄-INH and C4, and normal C3 value.* C1̄-INH function should then be tested in esterolytic assay, low values being highly indicative of HAE. The investigation of family members should help clarify the hereditary background and detect any further undisclosed cases. Cases have been described, however, where no evidence of heredity could be found despite strong indications of HAE in the patient who was thus the mutant [113]. C1q and C1 are usually normal in HAE, which helps distinguish it from the acquired form of C1̄-INH deficiency, where C1q and C1 values are low [20, 59].

2. *Highly increased value of C1̄-INH in the immunochemical test, low C4 and normal C3 values.* Type-2 HAE (table II) is to be suspected. C1̄-INH function should be investigated by esterolytic assay and if values are low crossed immunoelectrophoresis is recommended to check for the presence of the double-peaked C1̄-INH precipitates (fig. 3).

3. *Normal or slightly decreased value of C1̄-INH, low C4 and normal C3 values.* Variants of type 3 and 4 may be suspected; the finding of a non-functioning C1̄-INH in the esterolytic assay supports a diagnosis of HAE type-3; further investigations and a family study are necessary to confirm diagnosis.

Table II. Laboratory findings in HAE

HAE	$C\bar{1}$-INH			C4	C1q	C3
	rocket electro-phoresis	estero-lytic test[1] U/ml	inhibition of $C\bar{1}$ splitting activity on C4	immuno-chemical test %	immuno-chemical test %	immuno-chemical test %
Conventional form, type 1	<30	<6	no	<30	N	N
Variant form, type 2	>200	<6	no	<30	N	N
Variant form, type 3	100	<6	no	<30	N	N
Variant form, type 4	100	N	no	<30	N	N
Normal range, %	72–153	18–28		53–207		

N = Normal.

[1] According to *Laurell and Siboo* [93].

Where esterolytic assay gives normal $C\bar{1}$-INH values, but the clinical picture and anamnestic data indicate an inherited trait, further investigation will be necessary with functional analysis of the capacity of the patient's serum to inhibit $C\bar{1}$s splitting activity of C4 [146].

In the majority of cases where HAE is suspected, laboratory diagnosis is a simple and cheap procedure (HAE types 1 and 2). Extensive and more sophisticated analysis will only rarely be required – as, for example, where types 3 and 4, the two uncommon variants of HAE, cannot be excluded by screening tests, or where an immune complex disorder in HAE with consumption of C1q and C3 may complicate diagnosis.

Table I lists the tests used in the laboratory diagnosis of HAE, and table II shows the results of the analysis of HAE variants.

Therapy

Various therapeutic methods have been proposed for the prevention and control of HAE attacks. Early on it was reported that the intervals between attacks could be prolonged by giving methyltestosterone [14, 86, 163], but its use proved to be limited owing to the side effects arising in continuous therapy.

Although treatment with plasma transfusions has been reported to be successful [135], in some cases symptoms have been aggravated by plasma infusion, apparently owing to the supply of the substrates for C1 esterase, C4 and C2 [2].

ε-Aminocaproic acid (EACA) or tranexamic acid was found successful early in a few cases, inasmuch as attacks were prevented or reduced in severity, or the interval between them prolonged by continuous administration [21, 113, 127]. Further studies showed these drugs to be useful in about 80% of HAE patients [13, 24, 54, 155]; again, however, side effects occurred in some cases, while in others treatment failed to produce any effect at all, and even deterioration of symptoms was sometimes noted [77]. The therapeutic effect of EACA and tranexamic acid is probably due to their capacity to inhibit enzymes that are capable of activating C1, either directly, or indirectly by consumption of C$\bar{1}$-INH. In view of the physiological activation of C1 [96, 99, 102, 174, 175] and the increased C1 activation that may occur in various situations such as trauma and infection, it is reasonable to assume that EACA and tranexamic acid help to control the physiological activation of C1, as well as any accelerated C1 activation under conditions likely to give rise to attacks. The low level of C$\bar{1}$-INH ($<$ 30% of the normal) is apparently insufficient to contend with increased local activation of C1 in the tissues caused by infections, or release of proteolytic enzymes.

New drugs in the control of HAE were introduced with the synthetic attenuated anabolic androgens, danazol and stanazol, drugs with rather few side effects [60, 136, 144, 156]. After treatment most patients will be symptom-free, or at least the severity of their angioedema attacks is significantly reduced. Interestingly, the low level of 30% or less of the normal C$\bar{1}$-INH concentration in the type-1 group of HAE increases to 50–70%, and C4 and C2 values rapidly normalize. In healthy people, danazol administration causes a 50% increase of the C$\bar{1}$-INH, while the C4 level remains largely unchanged [60, 103], which explains the normalization of C$\bar{1}$-INH in HAE patients on danazol treatment. Like other anabolic steroids, danazol apparently affects the C$\bar{1}$-INH synthesizing liver cells (by specific receptors), triggering the functioning C$\bar{1}$-INH gene to increase its mRNA production. When the functioning C$\bar{1}$-INH increases to a critical level in the circulation and in the tissues, C1 activation will be controlled and consumption of C4 and C2 will be prevented, resulting in a rapid normalization of their concentrations.

In patients who do not respond to danazol or to tranexamic acid treatment, and in patients where suboptimal doses have to be used (as in children and in pregnant women) a combination of both drugs would seem to be a logical alternative [89]. Such an approach might also be motivated by the risk of hepatic damage and liver neoplasma caused by long-term treatment with androgen derivatives [52, 104, 172]. Even when no signs of liver damage were noted in 13 HAE patients treated with danazol in a follow-up study of between 15 and 48 months, the use of minimal effective doses was emphasized [25].

Intravenous administration of partially purified $C\bar{1}$-INH, used in 8 patients during acute laryngeal or abdominal attacks, resulted in mitigation of their symptoms and increase of C4 levels. Infusion of purified $C\bar{1}$-INH preparations has also been successfully used in severe, potentially fatal attacks [9, 24, 57], marked improvement being noted within 20–30 min after infusion and emergency tracheotomy was unnescessary. 30 severe attacks were promptly reversed by the use of $C\bar{1}$-INH infusion. Using a highly purified concentrate of $C\bar{1}$-INH, substitution has been sucessful also in preventing attacks [71].

Concluding Remarks on HAE

Earlier reports showed a high mortality rate in HAE (about 25%). Modern therapy has enabled patients to live normal lives and has impressively reduced the mortality rate. It is therefore of the utmost importance to recognize these patients, and diagnosis by the assays outlined above is relatively simple and well within the capacity of most immunological and clinical-chemical laboratories. Each new case should lead to screening of the patient's family to ensure the early detection of further potential or undisclosed cases.

The understanding of HAE as a genetic deficiency of $C\bar{1}$-INH without primary immunological disorders, and with secondary defects within the complement system including low concentrations of C4 and C2, with all other complement factors being within the normal range, has contributed to our knowledge of the biological role played by the complement system. The finding of an increased frequency of immune complex-related diseases, such as systemic lupus erythematosus-like syndromes, in HAE patients focuses attention on the chronically exhausted classical pathway as a possible pathogenetic factor in the development of immune complex diseases.

Knowledge of the mediator(s) in HAE is growing but remains fragmentary, and it will be essential to clarify controversial findings. The further development of chemical analysis of the variants of the C$\bar{1}$-INH, should contribute to an understanding of the biological disorder and the genetic background in HAE.

Acquired C$\bar{1}$-Inhibitor Deficiency with Angioedema and/or Urticaria

Association with Lymphoproliferative Disease

Caldwell et al. [20] reported on 2 patients with angioedema where low functional C$\bar{1}$-INH and low serum concentrations of C$\bar{1}$-INH were found. Both of them developed lymphosarcoma. Complement analysis revealed low C1, C2 and C4 values, but C3 was within the normal range. IgM was markedly increased, and in one of them a considerable amount of 7S IgM was present in serum. Circulating C1q-binding substances were not detected. Thus, the complement pattern found definitely distinguished this syndrome from HAE, where C1 activity is normal [18, 20]. Furthermore family studies failed to provide evidence of a hereditary trait.

Several other patients with these characteristics have since been described [42, 69, 70, 147, 157]. The distinction from HAE was clear: no hereditary trait was demonstrated, and the complement pattern differed from that found in HAE, as C1 and its subcomponents were decreased. In some of the patients, however, C3 was normal as in HAE, which may indicate a fluid phase activation of C1, C4 and C2 [20].

Common to all published cases belonging to this category are abnormalities of the immunoglobulins with the presence of monoclonal Ig populations of IgG or IgM classes, circulating cryoglobulins of IgG or IgM class, and in some cases antibodies to leucemic lymphocytes or to abnormal mononuclear cells.

A group of patients closely related to those with lymphoproliferative malignancy may be considered to be a special category. The same C disorder appears with low C$\bar{1}$-INH values obtained by functional and immunochemical tests, low C1 and C1 subcomponents, low concentrations of C4 and C2 and, in some cases, low C3 and C5. M-components of IgG or IgM classes were reported to be present in their circulation. Several of these patients suffered from angioedema and/or chronic urticaria or other seemingly allergic diseases [30, 59, 76, 95, 98, 129, 151]. Rectal carcinoma and angioedema were found in 1 patient [27].

We have followed one such patient for more than 8 years, using complement and other immunological analyses [91]. The patient, a male,

Table III. Complement analysis of samples from a patient with chronic urticaria and acquired C1̄-INH deficiency

Sample No.	C1̄-INH		Immunochemical complexes, %				
	rocket electro-phoresis %	esterolytic assay[1] U/ml	C1q	C1s	C3	C4	C1̄r-C1̄s-C1̄-INH
1	44	11	<5	38	10	4	high diffuse precipitates
2	58	11	3	53	14	6	high diffuse precipitates
3	50	16	7	< 5	14	4	high diffuse precipitates
4	55	10	<5	< 5	14	4	high diffuse precipitates
5	63	10	n.d.	n.d.	8	3	high diffuse precipitates
6	49	12	n.d.	n.d.	19	4	high diffuse precipitates
Normal range	72–153	18–28	78–130	79–149	70–136	53–207	

The results recorded are from samples obtained during a 2-year period. n.d. = Not done.
[1] According to *Laurell and Siboo* [93].

first appeared at the age of 35 years with severe cold urticaria. The disease has persisted without improvement despite various intensive attempts to deal with it, including treatment with tranexamic acid, danazol, and plasma transfusions. No signs of lymphoproliferative disease have been noted and no other immunologically related disease has developed. The analysis of the complement system and C1̄-INH is given in table III. The typical pattern with low C1̄-INH, measured functionally and immunochemically, low C1q, C4 and C3 were found, and C5 was also decreased. No signs of activation of the alternative pathway were found, as factor B and properdin were normal. C1̄r-C1̄s-C1̄-INH complexes were constantly present in high quantities. No circulating immune complexes have been found (as determined by the C1q-binding assay, the C1q deviation test or the solid phase assay). Tests for rheumatoid factors, antinuclear factors, and C1q precipitins have been negative. About 3 years after the onset of the symptoms the patient developed a discrete M component of IgG class with a concentration of about 1 g/l, which since then has remained fairly constant. It should be mentioned that the patient has an identical twin who

Table IV. C activation by purified, non-aggregated M-component from a patient with acquired C1̄-INH deficiency

	C1̄r-C1̄s-C1̄-INH %	C2 conversion	C3 conversion	C3d
Normal serum + purified M component	25	+	+	+
Normal serum + veronal-buffered saline	12	–	–	–
Normal serum + polyclonal IgG, not aggregated	12	–	–	–

Conversion of C2 and C3 was assessed by crossed immunoelectrophoresis.
C3d was measured by the method of *Johnson* [74].

is perfectly healthy and in whom no complement or immunoglobulin abnormality has been found. The results of further studies [109] on the effects on the C system of his M component in highly purified form and free from aggregates are given in table IV. On incubation of normal serum with the purified IgG component, the concentration of the C1̄r-C1̄s-C1̄-INH complexes were doubled, C2 and C3 were converted (studied by crossed immunoelectrophoresis) and C3d was formed. Hitherto, however, attempts to show binding of C1q to the non-aggregated IgG-M component have failed [*Lindgren,* personal commun.].

Other such cases of patients with severe edema without signs of malignancy or immunologically related diseases and with similar disorders of C1̄-INH and the complement system and presence of M components in serum have been reported. *Cicardi* et al. [23] presented 2 such cases, one of which, a middle aged male, had attacks of angioedema sometimes complicated with laryngeal edema. C analysis showed low C1̄-INH by functional and immunochemical assays and low concentrations of C1 and C4. 2 years after the onset of the disease a monoclonal IgM appeared in his serum. C1̄-INH turnover studies showed a markedly accelerated C1̄-INH consumption. Signs of proliferative disease were not demonstrated during an observation period of 5 years. Treatment with C1̄-INH concentrate during an acute attack of laryngeal edema followed by danazol for prophylactic purposes, was highly effective at first, but after 8 months the drug ceased to have any effect.

The $C\bar{1}$-INH turnover in healthy people and in HAE patients has been studied by *Quastel* et al. [139]. The fractional catabolic rate of $C\bar{1}$-INH was 2.5% in normals, and that in HAE patients 3.5% of the total body pool per hour. In contrast, in 6 patients with acquired $C\bar{1}$-INH deficiency, of whom 1 had an IgA-M component and another an IgM component, the fractional catabolic rate was 6% [*Rosen,* personal commun.]. It was also shown that the M components had no antibody-binding activity to $C\bar{1}$-INH, nor did they bind $C\bar{1}$-INH. The monoclonal M-component-producing cells, taken from blood or spleen, did not bind $C\bar{1}$-INH or C1 in excess of that observed in control B cells from patients with chronic lymphatic leukemia and no $C\bar{1}$-INH deficiency.

What is the primary disorder in this form of acquired $C\bar{1}$-INH deficiency remains an unanswered question. The increased turnover of $C\bar{1}$-INH [23; and *Rosen,* personal commun.] might be explained by complex formation with $C\bar{1}r$-$C\bar{1}s$ of the C1 complex after activation by C1-binding immune complexes or other activators. The low concentrations of C1 and its subcomponents, and of C2, C4 and C3 may be in keeping with increased activation of the cascade along the classical pathway, though C1q-binding immune complexes and other C1q-binding substances have not been shown in all cases. Such an interpretation is, however, not easily reconcilable with findings that, with rare exceptions, $C\bar{1}$-INH is usually normal or increased when measured both immunochemically and functionally in active SLE where high amounts of circulating immune complexes and intense activation of C1 are found [166]. Furthermore, in mixed cryoglobulinemia with low concentrations of C1, C4 and C2, the $C\bar{1}$-INH protein concentration and function was not found to be reduced in a study of 18 patients with hypocomplementemia [36]. An explanation of the binding and consumption of $C\bar{1}$-INH to constituents in plasma or to abnormal cells (lymphocytes?) resulting in an inability to regulate the physiological C1 activation seems unlikely in view of *Rosen's* findings (see above).

Acquired Angioedema with Decreased $C\bar{1}$-INH Function and Normal Amounts of $C\bar{1}$-INH Protein

On forming complex with kallikrein, $C\bar{1}$-INH loses its $C\bar{1}$-inhibiting function and the enzymatic activity of kallikrein is eliminated [63]. Immunochemical studies have shown that both proteins in the kallikrein-$C\bar{1}$-INH complex retain their antigenic capacity [5, 29].

In studies of large numbers of patients with chronic idiopathic urticaria and angioedema, disorders within the complement system were only rarely found [6, 98, 116]. Few deficiencies of the major plasma protease inhibitors were found in comprehensive studies of angioedema [51, 117], and when present their significance was difficult to evaluate [117]. In 150 patients with angioedema or chronic urticaria, concentrations of C$\bar{1}$-INH were found to be normal when measured by electroimmunoassay; in the functional test, however, they were low in 14 patients in whom no abnormality of the components of the classical pathway could be found [98].

One such patient, studied for many years both clinically and with C analysis [91], is a now 70-year-old female with a 17-year history of angioedema and episodic, painful joint symptoms classified as 'allergic arthritis'. Attacks were frequent, occurring every 10–14 days and lasting 1–3 days. Immunoglobulins were within the normal ranges, and no M components, circulating immune complexes, rheumatoid factors or antinuclear factors were found. During attacks the functional C$\bar{1}$-INH test showed low values, while immunochemically the values remained within the normal range. In symptom-free periods, C$\bar{1}$-INH activity was normal. Total hemolytic complement activity (CH_{50}) and functional hemolytic C4 tests showed normal values. C1 esterase activity was undetectable in fresh serum, but was generated by incubation for about 30 min or less at 37 °C in samples obtained during attacks, most probably reflecting the inability of the low-functioning C$\bar{1}$-INH to inhibit C1 activation. During a severe attack the patient was given plasma transfusion and treatment with Karbamezipin (Tegretol), after which she was symptom-free for nearly 2 years, during which C$\bar{1}$-INH function was normal. Relapse of her angioedema occurred 2 months after Tegretol had been discontinued and again C$\bar{1}$-INH function fell (table V). In order to investigate the possible effect of Tegretol on the synthesis of C$\bar{1}$-INH, samples from patients with epilepsy were obtained before, during and 14 days after treatment with Tegretol. No differences were noted in the concentrations of C$\bar{1}$-INH in the immunochemical or functional tests, excluding any direct synthesis-inducing effect of Tegretol.

Thus in this patient functional C$\bar{1}$-INH tests showed fluctuating values with about 6–8 U/ml (normal 18–28 U/ml) during attacks, but normal amounts of C$\bar{1}$-INH protein and no abnormalities of the components of the classical pathway or total hemolytic complement activity were recorded. The suspicion that activation of the kallikren system was

Table V. $C\bar{1}$-INH in a patient with angioedema associated with fluctuating function of $C\bar{1}$-INH

Sample No.	$C\bar{1}$-INH		Disease activity
	immunochemical %	functional U/ml	
1	68	6	angioedema
2	90	13	angioedema
3	114	20	symptom-free
4	93	3	angioedema
5	n.d.	18	symptom-free
6	n.d.	10	angioedema
7	95	9	angioedema
8	n.d.	19	symptom-free
9	146	26	severe joint symptoms
Normal range	72–153	18–28	

CH_{50} and functional tests for C4 were normal. The analyses recorded were performed on samples obtained during a 5-year period. n.d. = Not done.

involved could not be verified, however. Thus no consumption of prekallikrein or presence of kallikrein-like activity was noted using a recently developed chromogenic substrate method [58] (AB Kabi Diagnostica, Sweden). The background of the disease in this patient is not clear.

Colman et al. [29] described patients with typhoid fever with normal values in immunochemical tests but low concentrations of functional $C\bar{1}$-INH, which returned to the normal when the infection was cured. The reduced function of $C\bar{1}$-INH was caused by activation of kallikrein and complex formation with $C\bar{1}$-INH. No information was given on symptoms of angioedema in conjunction with the reduced $C\bar{1}$-INH function, or on the complement profile.

Several other patients with long-standing angioedema and similar $C\bar{1}$-INH disorders but normal complement function, have been observed in our laboratory for extended follow-up periods.

Table VI. Laboratory findings in angioedema or chronic urticaria associated with C$\bar{1}$-INH abnormality

	HAE conventional form	HAE variant forms	Acquired C$\bar{1}$-INH deficiency[1]	
			1	2
HIG assay				
Classical pathway	abnornal	abnormal	abnormal	normal
Alternative pathway	normal	normal	normal or abnormal	normal
C$\bar{1}$-INH				
Immunochemical test	low	high or normal	low	normal
Functional test	low	low	low	low
C4	low	low	low	normal
C1q	normal	normal	low	normal

HIG = Hemolysis in gel assay.
[1] 1 and 2 refer to the description in the text of acquired C$\bar{1}$-INH deficiency.

Laboratory Diagnosis in Acquired C$\bar{1}$-INH Deficiency

Complement screening for this disease includes simple hemolysis in gel techniques for the classical and alternative pathways [171], immunochemical measurement of C1q and C4, and immunochemical and functional testing of C$\bar{1}$-INH.

1. Low levels of C$\bar{1}$-INH protein, C1q and C4 combined with low C$\bar{1}$-INH activity, favor this diagnosis, which is further supported if an M component is present. C3 may be low or normal and decreased C activity in the HIG test for the classical pathway is noted (table VI).

2. Normal values of C$\bar{1}$-INH, C1q and C4 in the immunochemical assays, and normal C activity in the HIG tests, but decreased C$\bar{1}$-INH function measured by the esterolytic assay or the immunochemical functional assay [180], indicate disorders primarily of enzyme systems outside the C system. Estimation of activation of kallikrein may be the next step in the investigation [58] (table VI).

Distinction between HAE and Acquired C1̄-INH Deficiency Based on Laboratory Analysis

Low values obtained by immunochemical and functional C1̄-INH assays do not discriminate between the two conditions; nor does C4 analysis as C4 is low in all HAE cases and in some cases of acquired deficiency. A normal C4 concentration, however, precludes a HAE diagnosis. Both C1 and C1q are virtually normal in HAE, which distinguishes it from certain of the acquired forms. The inclusion of the immunochemical functional C1̄-INH assay, described by *Ziccardi and Cooper* [180], among the tests probably ensures the detection of acquired C1̄-INH deficiency with non-functioning but immunochemically reactive inhibitor, as well as of the conventional and variant forms of HAE. A combination of laboratory analysis to distinguish between the various forms of HAE and the acquired C1̄-INH deficiencies is proposed in table VI.

Angioedema and/or Urticaria in Conjunction with Abnormal Complexes of C1 Subcomponents and C1̄-INH

In a study of 150 patients with angioedema and/or urticaria, abnormal complexes of C1r-C1s in proenzyme form were found in sera from 11% of the patients, and signs of C1 activation – with pathologically increased concentrations of C1̄r-C1̄s-C1̄-INH complexes – in 33% [98].

Disorders of the C1 subcomponents that occur in certain cases of angioedema and/or urticaria can be detected by crossed immunoelectrophoresis (fig. 4). The cause and significance of the formation of the proenzyme C1r-C1s complexes is not known, it might indicate an increased consumption of C1q after its release from the synthesizing cells, before the extracellular complexing with C1r-C1s takes place. Another possibility might be an imbalance in the synthesis of C1q and of C1r-C1s, their concentrations normally being highly correlated [98]. It is also possible that substances, capable of binding C1q in the C1qrs complex without activating C1r-C1s, exist in the tissues and the circulation [111], and may produce a shift in the dissociation equilibrium of the C1qrs complex and a consequent surplus of C1r-C1s [7, 119].

The increased amounts of C1̄r-C1̄s-C1̄-INH complexes frequently found in this study strongly suggest the pathogenic significance of activation of C1 and the classical pathway [98]. An increase of C1̄r-C1̄s-C1̄-INH complexes is a sensitive indicator of C1 activation [10, 35, 64, 100]. The

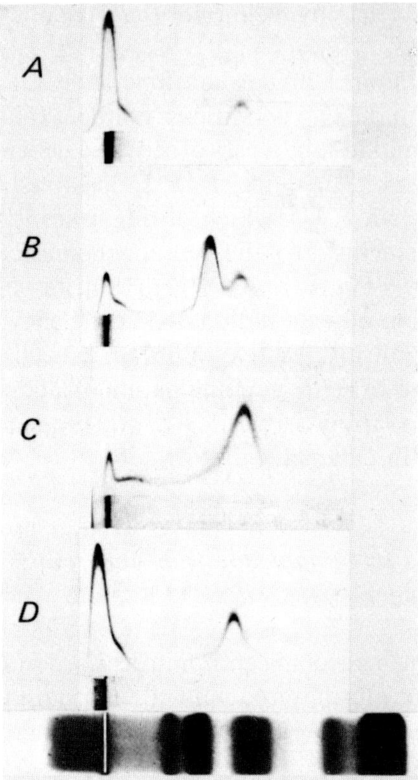

Fig. 4. Demonstration by crossed immunoelectrophoresis of complexes of $C\bar{1}r$-$C\bar{1}s$-$C\bar{1}$-INH and proenzyme C1r-C1s. *A* Normal serum. *B, C, D* Sera from patients with angioedema and urticaria. Both electrophoretic steps were run in Ca^{2+} containing buffer. Anti-C1s was added to the agarose gel in the secondary electrophoretic step [from ref. 98, with permission].

methods hitherto most commonly used in large scale investigations to estimate activation and consumption of the factors of both the classical pathway and the alternative pathway are rather crude instruments. The broad normal ranges of the concentrations of the complement factors and the fact that several of them behave as acute phase protein with increased synthesis during inflammation will tend to conceal the consumption and to complicate analysis. In addition to the measurement of $C\bar{1}r$-$C\bar{1}s$-$C\bar{1}$-INH complexes, recently developed methods for determining fragments of

C2 [164], C3 [17, 74, 165], and C4 [120] will improve the possibility of evaluating complement disorders in angioedema in relation to the pathogenesis and the disease state.

Concluding Remarks

Among patients with long-standing angioedema there are subjects with a non-hereditary disorder of $C\bar{1}$-INH, combined with consumption of the components of the classical C pathway, which are often associated with lymphoproliferative malignancy or diseases with an immunological background. Whether the $C\bar{1}$-INH and the complement disorders are the primary events or the results of other factors, for instance in malignancy, is not yet clear. In some of these patients, however, malignancy within the lymphatic system was not a prerequisite of the acquired $C\bar{1}$-INH deficiency.

Among patients with deviating $C\bar{1}$-INH values, obtained by immunochemical or functional analysis, and with normal patterns of the C factors of the classical pathway, activation ot other enzyme systems with consumption of $C\bar{1}$-INH may be involved.

It is possible that activation of the kallikrein or complement systems, or both, are involved in the pathogenesis of angioedema more often than studies of the concentrations of $C\bar{1}$-INH and other protease inhibitors would seem to indicate. Since the pathological process with activation and complex formation with inhibitors occurs in the intercellular space, it is quite possible that the complex formed between the activated enzymes and available inhibitors will be eliminated before they reach the circulation, and that feedback synthesis compensates for the consumption of the components composing the enzyme-inhibitor complexes, such as kallikrein-$C\bar{1}$-INH and $C\bar{1}$r-$C\bar{1}$s-$C\bar{1}$-INH complexes. Analogy with other fields might indicate this to be the cause of the normal values often encountered in serum and plasma in angioedema, where activation of C or kallikrein, or both, may have occurred. Thus in rheumatoid arthritis a pronounced activation of the early C components of the classical pathway occurs in the joints, while in most patients their concentrations in serum and plasma remain within normal ranges or are even increased [10, 112, 126, 150]. Another example is acute pancreatitis, where the concentrations of most of the protease inhibitors in plasma are often normal, while clear changes of the inhibitor patterns are found in samples from lymph vessels draining the pancreas and in the peritoneal fluid – changes dependent on binding to liberated pancreatic enzymes. Only in severe cases is inhibitor consumption obvious in the circulation [131].

Further Aspects on Angioedema

A few reports are available which may point to a relationship between angioedema and defects of regulators within the C system, other than $C\bar{1}$-INH. In the patient first described with factor-I deficiency, in addition to the infections dominating the clinical picture, angioedema was observed after he had taken a hot shower [1].

A patient with abnormally low amounts of the anaphylatoxin inactivator, carboxypeptidase N, suffered from angioedema [118], the values for anaphylatoxin inactivator being 50% of normal, possibly indicating a recessive hereditary trait. 1 healthy sibling, however, had a similarly low concentration of anaphylatoxin inactivator, which may indicate that other, unknown factors also contribute to the predisposition to angioedema.

References

1 Alper, C.A.; Abramson, N.; Johnston, R.B., Jr.; Jandl, J.H.; Rosen, F.S.: Increased susceptibility to infection associated with abnormalities of complement-mediated functions and of the third component of complement (C3). New Engl. J. Med. *282:* 349–354 (1970).

2 Alper, C.A.; Rosen, F.S.: Genetics of the complement system. Adv. hum. Genet. *7:* 141–188 (1976).

3 Arlaud, G.J.; Reboul, A.; Sim, R.B.; Colomb, M.G.: Interaction of $C\bar{1}$ inhibitor with $C\bar{1}r$ and $C\bar{1}s$ subcomponents in human $C\bar{1}$. Biochim. biophys. Acta *576:* 151–162 (1979).

4 Axelsson, U.; Laurell, A.-B.: A case of angioneurotic edema with a high content of non-functioning, double peaked C1 esterase inhibitor. Clin. exp. Immunol. *8:* 511–516 (1970).

5 Bagdasarian, A.; Biswajit, L.; Talamo, R.C.; Wong, P.; Colman, R.: Immunochemical studies of plasma kallikrein. J. clin. Invest. *54:* 1444–1454 (1974).

6 Ballow, M.; Ward, G.W.; Gershwin, M.E.; Day, N.K.: C1-bypass complement activation pathway in patients with chronic urticaria and angioedema. Lancet *ii:* 248–250 (1975).

7 Bartholomew, R.M.; Esser, A.F.: The first complement component: evidence for an equilibrium between C1s free in serum and C1s bound in the C1 complex. J. Immun. *119:* 1916–1922 (1977).

8 Becker, E.L.: Nature and classification of immediate-type allergic reactions. Adv. Immunol. *13:* 307–308 (1971).

9 Bergamaschini, L.; Tucci, A.; Gardinali, M.; Frangi, D.; Valle, C.; Agostoni, A.: Replacement therapy in acute attacks of HAE with C1̄ inhibitor (C1̄ INH) concentrate. Int. Conf. 'Clinical aspects of complement mediated diseases', Bellagio 1983, p. 31.

10 Berglund, K.; Laurell, A.-B; Nived, O.; Sjöholm, A.G.; Sturfelt, G.: Complement activation, circulating C1q binding substances and inflammatory activity in rheumatoid arthritis. Relations and changes on suppression of inflammation. J. clin. lab. Immunol. *4:* 7–14 (1980).

11 Betz, S.J.; Isliker, H.: Antibody-independent interactions between *Escherichia coli* 15 and human complement components. J. Imun. *127:* 1748–1754 (1981).

12 Bhakdi, S.; Tranum-Jensen, J.: Molecular nature of the complement lesion. Proc. natn Acad. Sci. USA *75:* 5655–5659 (1978).

13 Blohmé, G.: Treatment of hereditary angioneurotic edema with tranexamic acid. A random double-blind cross-over study. Acta med. scand. *192:* 293–298 (1972).

14 Blohmé, G.; Ysander, L.; Korsan-Bengtsen, K.; Laurell, A.-B.: Hereditary angioneurotic edema in three families. Symptomatic heterogeneity, complement analysis and therapeutic trials. Acta med. scand. *191:* 209–219 (1971).

15 Bokisch, V.A.; Müller-Eberhard, H.J.; Cochrane, C.G.: Isolation of a fragment (C3a) of the third component of human complement containing anaphylatoxin and chemotactic activity and description of an anaphylatoxin inactivator of human serum. J. exp. Med. *129:* 1109–1130 (1969).

16 Bourgarit, J.J.; Lopez-Trascasa, M.; Moisy, M.; Sobel, A.T.: Identification of C2k, a C2 derived vasoactive peptide. Fed. Proc. *42:* 1234 (1983).

17 Brandslund, I.; Siersted, H.C.; Svehag, S.-E.; Teisner, B.: Double-decker rocket-immunoelectrophoresis for direct quantitition of complement split products with C3d specificity in plasma. J. immunol. Methods *44:* 63–71 (1981).

18 Brecy, H.; Hartmann, L.: Distinction between hereditary and acquired angioneurotic angioedema according to the complement system. Biomedicine *23:* 328–334 (1975).

19 Budzko, D.B.; Müller-Eberhard, H.J.: Cleavage of the fourth component of human complement (C4) by C1 esterase: isolation and characterization of the low molecular weight product. Immunochemistry *7:* 227–234 (1970).

20 Caldwell, J.R.; Ruddy, S.; Schur, P.H.; Austen, K.F.: Acquired C1̄ inhibitor deficiency in lymphosarcoma. Clin. Immunol. Immunopathol. *1:* 39–52 (1972).

21 Champion, R.H.; Lachmann, P.J.: Hereditary angioedema treated with ε-aminocaproic acid. Br. J. Derm. *81:* 763–765 (1969).

22 Chesne, S.; Villiers, C.L.; Arlaud, G.J.; Lacroix, M.B.; Colomb, M.G.: Fluid phase interaction of C1̄ inhibitor (C1̄ INH) and the subcomponents C1̄r and C1̄s of the first component of complement. Biochem. J. *201:* 61–70 (1982).

23 Cicardi, M.; Bergamaschini, L.; Tucci, A.; Valle, C.: Uninherited C1̄ INH deficiency with angioedema symptoms. Report of two cases. Int. Conf. 'Clinical aspects of complement mediated diseases', Bellagio 1983, p. 36.

24 Cicardi, M.; Bergamaschini, L.; Marasini, B.; Boccasini, G.; Tucci, A.; Agostoni, A.: Hereditary angioedema: an appraisal of 104 cases. Am. J. med. Sci. *284:* 2–9 (1982).

25 Cicardi, M.; Bergamaschini, L.; Tucci, A.; Agostoni, A.; Tornaghi, G.; Cocci, G.; Colombi, R.; Viale, G.: Morphologic evaluation of the liver in hereditary angioedema patients on long-term treatment with androgen derivates. J. Allergy clin. Immunol. *72:* 294–298 (1983).

26 Claus, D.R.; Siegel, J.; Petras, K.; Osmand, A.P.; Gewurz, H.: Interaction of C-reactive protein with the first component of human complement. J. Immun. *119:* 187–192 (1977).

27 Cohen, S.H.; Koethe, S.M.; Kozin, F.; Rodey, G.; Arkins, J.A.; Fink, J.N.: Acquired angioedema associated with rectal carcinoma and its response to danazol therapy. J. Allergy clin. Immunol. *62:* 217–221 (1978).

28 Collen, D.: Identification and some properties of a new fast-reacting plasmin inhibitor in human plasma. Eur. J. Biochem. *69:* 200–209 (1976).

29 Colman, R.W.; Edelman, R.; Scott, C.F.; Gilman, R.H.: Plasma kallikrein activation and inhibition during typhoid fever. J. clin. Invest. *61:* 287–296 (1978).

30 Constanzi, J.J.; Coltman, C.A.: Kappa chain cold precipitable immunoglobulin G (IgG) associated with cold urticaria. I. Clinical observations. Clin. exp. Immunol. *2:* 167–178 (1967).

31 Cooper, N.R.: Isolation and analysis of the mechanism of action of an inactivator of C4b in normal human serum. J. exp. Med. *141:* 890–903 (1975).

32 Cooper, N.R.; Jensen, F.C.; Welsh, R.M., Jr.; Oldstone, M.B.A.: Lysis of RNA tumor viruses by human serum: direct antibody independent triggering of the classical complement pathway. J. exp. Med. *144:* 970–984 (1976).

33 Cooper, N.R.; Morrison, D.C.: Binding and activation of the first component of complement by the lipid A region of lipopolysaccharides. J. Immun. *120:* 1862–1868 (1978).

34 Cooper, N.R.; Müller-Eberhard, H.J.: The reaction mechanism of human C5 in immune hemolysis. J. exp. Med. *132:* 775–793 (1970).

35 Cooper, N.R.; Nemerow, G.R.; Mayes, J.T.: Methods to detect and quantitate complement activation. Springer Semin, Immunopathol. *6:* 195–212 (1983).

36 Corvetta, A.; Spaeth, P.J.; Nydegger, U.E.: Does it exist an acquired $C\bar{1}$ inhibitor functional deficiency in essential mixed cryoglobulinemia? Int. Conf. 'Clinical aspects of complement mediated diseases', Bellagio 1983, p. 45.

37 Craddock, P.R.; Hammerschmidt, D.; White, J.G.; Dalmasso, A.P.; Jacob, H.S.: Complement (C5a) induced granulocyte aggregation in vitro. A possible mechanism of complement mediated leukostasis and leukopenia. J. clin. Invest. *60:* 260–264 (1977).

38 Curd, J.G.; Prograis, J.J., Jr.; Cochrane, C.G.: Detection of active kallikrein in induced blister fluids of hereditary angioedema patients. J. exp. Med. *152:* 742–747 (1980).

39 Curd, J.G.; Yelvington, M.; Burridge, N.; Strimler, N.P.; Gerard, C.; Prograis, L.J., Jr.; Cochrane, C.G.; Müller-Eberhard, H.J.: Generation of bradykinin during incubation of hereditary angioedema plasma. Mol. Immunol. *19:* 1365 (1982).

40 Damerau, B.; Vogt, W.: Pseudoallergic reactions based on effects of complement derived peptides on circulating leukocytes; in Dukor, Kallós, Schlumberges, West. PAR, pseudoallergic reactions, vol. 3, pp. 101–121 (Karger, Basel 1982).

41 Davis, A.E.; Davis, J.S.; Rabson, A.R.; Osofsky, S.G.; Colten, H.R.; Rosen, F.S.; Alper, C.A.: Homozygous C3 deficiency: detection of C3 by radioimmunoassay. Clin. Immunol. Immunopathol. *8:* 543–550 (1977).

42 Day, N.K.; Winfield, J.F.; Winchester, R.J.; Gee, T.S.; Kunkel, H.G.: Evidence for immune complexes involving antilymphocyte antibodies associated with hypocomplementemia in chronic lymphocytic leukemia (CLL). Clin. Res. *23:* 410 (1975).

43 Donaldson, V.H.: The challenge of hereditary angioneurotic edema. New Engl. J. Med. *308:* 1094–1095 (1983).

44 Donaldson, V.H.; Evans, R.R.: A biochemical abnormality in hereditary angioneurotic edema: absence of serum inhibitor of C1 esterase. Am. J. Med. *35:* 37–44 (1963).

45 Donaldson, V.H.; Rosen, F.S.: Action of complement in hereditary angioneurotic edema plasma. The role of C1 esterase. J. clin. Invest. *43:* 2204–2213 (1964).

46 Donaldson, V.H.; Rosen, F.S.: Hereditary angioneurotic edema. A clinical survey. Pediatrics, Springfield *37:* 1017–1027 (1966).

47 Donaldson, V.H.; Hess, E.W.; McAdams, A.J.: Lupus erythematosus-like disease in three unrelated women with hereditary angioneurotic edema. Ann. intern. Med. *86:* 312–313 (1977).

48 Donaldson, V.H.; Rosen, F.S.; Bing, D.H.: Role of second component of complement (C2) and plasmin in kinin release in hereditary angioneurotic edema. Trans. Ass. Am. Physns *90:* 174–183 (1977).

49 Donaldson, V.H.; Ratnoff, O.D.; Da Silva, W.D.; Rosen, F.S.: Permeability increasing activity in hereditary angioneurotic edema plasma. II. Mechanism of formation and partial characterization. J. clin. Invest. *48:* 642–653 (1969).

50 Dukor, P.; Kallós, P.; Schlumberger, H.D.; West, G.B.: PAR: pseudoallergic reactions. Involvement of drugs and chemicals; in Dukor, Kallós, Schlumberger, West, PAR, pseudoallergic reactions, pp. IX-IXV (Karger, Basel 1980).

51 Eftekhari, N.; Ward, A.M.; Allen, R.; Greaves, M.W.: Protease inhibitor profiles in urticaria and angioedema. Br. J. Derm. *101:* 17–20 (1979).

52 Farrel, G.G.; Joshua, V.E.; Uren, R.F.; Baird, P.J.; Perkins, R.W.; Kronenberg, H.: Androgen induced hepatoma. Lancet *i:* 430–432 (1975).

53 Fearon, D.T.; Austen, K.F.: Immunochemistry of the classical and alternative pathways of complement; in Glynn, Steward. Immunochemistry: an advanced textbook, pp. 365–397 (Wiley, New York 1978).

54 Forbes, C.D.; Pensky, J.; Ratnoff, O.D.: Inhibition of activated Hageman factor and activated plasma thromboplastin antecedent by purified C1 inactivator. J. Lab. clin. Med. *76:* 809–815 (1970).

55 Frank, M.M.; Sergent, J.S.; Kane, M.A.; Alling, D.W.: Epsilon aminocaproic acid therapy of hereditary angioneurotic edema: a double-blind study. New Engl. J. Med. *286:* 808–812 (1972).

56 Fritz, H.; Wunderer, G.; Kummer, K.; Heimburger, N.; Werle, E.: α_1-Antitrypsin und $C\bar{1}$ Inactivator. Progressive Inhibitoren für Serumkallikreine von Mensch und Schwein. Hoppe-Seyler's Z. physiol. Chem. *353:* 906–910 (1972).

57 Gadek, J.E.; Hosea, S.W.; Gelfand, J.A.; Santaella, M.; Wickerhauser, M.; Triantaphyllopoulos, D.C.; Frank, M.M.: Replacement therapy in hereditary angioedema. Successful treatment of acute episodes of angioedema with partly purified $C\bar{1}$ inhibitor. New Engl. J. Med. *302:* 542–546 (1980).

58 Gallimore, M.J.; Friberger, P.: Simple chromogenic peptide substrate assays for determining prekallikrein, kallikrein inhibition and kallikrein-like activity in human plasma. Thromb. Res. *25:* 293–298 (1982).

59 Gelfand, J.A.; Boss, C.R.; Conley, C.L.; Reinhart, R.; Frank, M.M.: Acquired C1 esterase inhibitor deficiency and angioedema. A review. Medicine, Baltimore *58:* 321–328 (1979).

60 Gelfand, J.A.; Sherings, R.J.; Alling, D.W.; Frank, M.M.: Treatment of hereditary angioedema with Danazol. Reversal of clinical and biochemical abnormalities. New Engl. J. Med. *295:* 1444–1448 (1976).

61 Gigli, I.; Austen, K.F.: Fluid phase destruction of $C2^{hu}$ by $C1^{hu}$. I. Its enhancement and inhibition by homologous and heterologous C4. J. exp. Med. *129:* 679–696 (1969).
62 Gigli, I.; Ruddy, S.; Austen, K.F.: The stoichometric measurement of the serum inhibitor of the first component of complement by the inhibition of immune hemolysis. J. Immun. *100:* 1154–1168 (1968).
63 Gigli, I.; Mason, J.W.; Colman, R.W.; Austen, K.F.: Interaction of plasma kallikrein with the $C\bar{1}$ inhibitor. J. Immun. *104:* 575–581 (1970).
64 Hack, C.E.; Hannema, A.J.; Eerenberg-Belmer, A.J.; Out, A.T.; Aalberse, R.C.: A $C\bar{1}$ inhibitor complex assay (INCA): a method to detect C1 activation in vitro and in vivo. J. Immun. *127:* 1450–1453 (1981).
65 Harpel, P.C.: Human plasma α_2-macroglobulin. An inhibitor of plasma kallikrein. J. exp. Med. *132:* 329–352 (1970).
66 Harpel, P.C.; Cooper, N.R.: Studies on plasma $C\bar{1}$ inactivator – enzyme interactions. I. Mechanism of interaction with $C\bar{1}$s, plasmin and trypsin. J. clin. Invest. *55:* 593–604 (1975).
67 Harpel, P.C.; Hugli, T.E.; Cooper, N.R.: Studies on plasma $C\bar{1}$ inactivator-enzyme interactions. II. Structural features of an abnormal $C\bar{1}$ inactivator from a kindred with hereditary angioneurotic edema. J. clin. Invest. *55:* 605–611 (1975).
68 Haupt, H.; Heimburger, N.; Krantz, T.; Schwick, H.G.: Ein Beitrag zur Isolierung und Charakterisierung des C1-Inaktivators aus Humanplasma. Eur. J. Biochem. *17:* 254–261 (1970).
69 Hauptmann, G.; Lang, J.M.; North, M.L.; Oberling, F.; Mayer, G.; Lachmann, P.J.: Acquired $C\bar{1}$ inhibitor deficiencies in lymphoproliferative diseases with serum immunoglobulin abnormalities. A study of three cases. Blut *32:* 195–206 (1976).
70 Hauptmann, G.; Mayer, S.; Lang, M.M.; Oberling, F.; Mayer, G.: Treatment of acquired $C\bar{1}$ inhibitor deficiency with danazol. Ann. intern. Med. *87:* 577–578 (1977).
71 Heimburger, N.; Pelzer, H.; Herber, H.; Preis, H.M.; Karges, H.E.: A highly purified concentrate of $C\bar{1}$ inhibitor for clinical use, which is heated in solution. Int. Conf. 'Clinical aspects of complement mediated diseases', Bellagio 1983, p. 33.
72 Hugli, T.E.; Müller-Eberhard, H.J.: Anaphylatoxins: C3a and C5a. Adv. Immunol. *26:* 1–53 (1978).
73 Jacob, H.S.; Craddock, P.R.; Hammerschmidt, E.E. Moldow, C.F.: Complement induced granulocyte aggregation. New Engl. J. Med. *302:* 789–794 (1980).
74 Johnson, U.: Influence of ageing and polyethyleneglycol on the quantitation of C3d in serum and plasma. Acta pathol. microbiol. scand., C, Immunol. (in press, 1984).
75 Johnson, A.M.; Alper, C.A.; Rosen, F.S.; Craig, J.M.: C1 inhibitor: evidence for decreased hepatic synthesis in hereditary angioneurotic edema. Science *173:* 553–554 (1971).
76 Jordon, R.E.; Duffie, F.C.; Good, R.A.; Day, N.K.; Diffuse normolipaemic plane xanthomatosis. An abnormal complement component profile. Clin. exp. Immunol. *18:* 407–415 (1974).
77 Juhlin, L.; Michaelsson, G.: Vascular reactions in hereditary angioneurotic edema. Acta derm.-vener., Stockh. *49:* 20–25 (1969).
78 Kagen, L.J.; Becker, E.L.: Inhibition of permeability globulin by C'1 esterase inhibitor. Fed. Proc. *22:* 613 (1963).

79 Kallós, P.; West, G.B.W.: Pseudo-allergic reactions in man; in Recent advances in clinical pharmacology, pp. 235–252 (Churchill Livingstone, Edinburgh 1983).

80 Kaplan, M.H.; Volanakis, J.E.: Interaction of C-reactive protein complexes with the complement system. I. Consumption of human complement associated with the reaction of C-reactive protein with pneumococcal C-polysaccharide and with choline phosphatides, lecithin and sphingomyelin. J. Immun. *112:* 2135–2147 (1974).

81 Kazatschkine, M.D.; Nydegger, U.E.: The human alternative complement pathway. Biology and immunopathology of activation and regulation. Prog. Allergy, vol. 30, pp. 193–234 (Karger, Basel 1982).

82 Klemperer, M.R.; Donaldson, V.H.; Rosen, F.S.: Effects of C′1 esterase on vascular permeability in man: studies in normal and complement deficient individuals and in patients with hereditary angioneurotic edema. J. clin. Invest. *47:* 604–611 (1968).

83 Klemperer, M.R.; Rosen, F.S.; Donaldson, V.H.: A polypeptide derived from the second component of complement (C2) which increases vascular permeability. J. clin. Invest. *48:* 44A (1969).

84 Kohler, P.F.; Percy, J.; Campion, V.M.; Smyth, C.: Hereditary angioedema and familial lupus erythematosus in identical twin boys. Am. J. Med. *56:* 406–411 (1974).

85 Kolb, W.P.; Müller-Eberhard, H.J.: Mode of action of human C9: adsorption of multiple C9 molecules to cellbound C8. J. Immun. *113:* 479–488 (1974).

86 Korsan-Bengtsen, K.; Ysander, L.; Blohmé, G.; Tibblin, E.: Extensive muscle necrosis after long-term treatment with ε-aminocaproic acid (EACA) in a case of hereditary angioneurotic edema. Acta med. scand. *185:* 341–346 (1969).

87 Lachmann, P.J.; Müller-Eberhard, H.J.: The demonstration in human serum of 'conglutinogen-activating factor' and its effect on the third component of complement. J. Immun. *100:* 691–698 (1968).

88 Lachmann, P.J.; Peters, D.K.: Complement; in Lachmann, Peters, Clinical aspects of immunology; 4th ed., pp. 18–49 (Blackwell Scientific, Oxford, 1980).

89 Lachmann, P.J.; Rosen, F.S.: Genetic defects of complement in man. Springer Semin. Immunpathol. *1:* 339–353 (1978).

90 Landerman, N.S.; Webster, M.E.; Becker, E.L.; Ratcliffe, H.E.: Hereditary angioneurotic edema: Deficiency of inhibitor for serum globulin permeability factor and/or plasma kallikrein. J. Allergy *33:* 330–341 (1962).

91 Laurell, A.-B.; Acquired $C\bar{1}$ inhibitor deficiency. Int. Conf. 'Clinical aspects of complement mediated diseases', Bellagio 1983, p. 35.

92 Laurell, A.-B.; Mårtensson, U.: $C\bar{1}$ inhibitor complexed with albumin in plasma from a patient with angioneurotic edema. Eur. J. Immunol. *1:* 146–149 (1971).

93 Laurell, A.-B.; Siboo, R.: Activation of C′1 to C′1 esterase on gel filtration on Sephadex G 200. Acta path. microbiol. scand. *68:* 230–242 (1966).

94 Laurell, A.-B.; Lund, B.; Malmquist, J.: Inability of highly purified streptokinase preparation to inactivate complement in serum. Acta path. microbiol. scand. *64:* 318–328 (1965).

95 Laurell, A.-B.; Mårtensson, U.; Sjöholm, A.G.: Complement components in hereditary angioedema and chronic urticaria. Int. Archs Allergy appl. Immunol. *49:* 86–88 (1975).

96 Laurell, A.-B.; Mårtensson, U.; Sjöholm, A.G.: C1 subcomponent complexes in normal and pathological sera studied by crossed immunoelectrophoresis. Acta pathol. microbiol. scand., B, Microbiol. *84:* 455–464 (1976).

97 Laurell, A.-B.; Mårtensson, U.; Sjöholm, A.G.: Electroimmunoassay of C1̄ inactivator and C4 in hereditary angioneurotic edema (HANE). Clin. Immunol. Immunopathol. *5:* 308–313 (1976).

98 Laurell, A.-B.; Mårtensson, U.; Sjöholm, A.G.: Studies of C1 subcomponents in chronic urticaria and angioedema. Int. Archs Allergy appl. Immunol. *54:* 434–442 (1977).

99 Laurell, A.-B.; Mårtensson, U.; Sjöholm, A.G.: Quantitation of C1̄r-C1̄s-C1̄ inactivator complexes by electroimmunoassay. Acta pathol. microbiol. scand., C, Immunol. *87:* 79–81 (1979).

100 Laurell, A.-B.; Johnson, U.; Mårtensson, U.; Sjöholm, A.G.: Formation of complexes of C1̄r, C1̄s and C1̄ inactivator in human sera on activation of C1. Acta pathol. microbiol. scand., C, Immunol. *86:* 299–306 (1978).

101 Laurell, A.-B.; Lindegren, J.; Malmros, I.; Mårtensson, H.: Enzymatic and immunochemical estimation of C1 esterase inhibitor in sera from patients with hereditary angioneurotic edema. Scand. J. clin. Lab. Invest. *24:* 221–225 (1969).

102 Laurell, A.-B.; Sjöholm, A.G.; Johnson, U.; Mårtensson, U.: Circulating complexes between C1r and C1s and between C1̄r, C1̄s and C1̄ inactivator; in Opferkuch, Rother, Schultz, Clinical aspects of the complement system, pp. 21–26 (Thieme, Stuttgart 1978).

103 Laurell, C.-B.; Rannevik, G.: A comparison of plasma protein changes induced by danazol, pregnancy and estrogens. J. clin. Endocr. Metab. *49:* 719–725 (1979).

104 Leonard-Johnson, F.; Lerner, K.G.; Siegel, M.; Feagler, J.R.; Majerus, P.W.; Hartmann, J.R.; Thomas, E.D.: Association of androgenic-anabolic steroid therapy with development of hepatocellular carcinoma. Lancet *ii:* 1273–1276 (1972).

105 Lepow, I.H.: Permeability-producing peptide byproduct of the interaction of the first, fourth and second component of complement; in Austen, Becker, Biochemistry of acute allergic reactions, pp. 205–215 (Blackwell, Oxford 1971).

106 Lepow, I.H.; Ratnoff, O.D.; Levy, L.R.: Studies on the activation of a proesterase associated with partially purified first component of complement. J. exp. Med. *107:* 451–474 (1958).

107 Lepow, I.H.; Naff, G.B.; Todd, E.W.; Pensky, J.; Hintz, C.F.: Chromatographic resolution of the first component of complement into three activities. J. exp. Med. *117:* 983–1008 (1963).

108 Levy, L.R.; Lepow, I.H.: Assay and properties of serum inhibitor of C′1 esterase. Proc. Soc. exp. Biol. Med. *101:* 608–611 (1959).

109 Lindgren, S.; Johnson, U.; Sjöholm, A.G.: Laurell, A.-B.: Studies on acquired C1̄ inhibitor deficiency: Effect on C factors of the isolated M-component from patient's serum (to be published).

110 Loos, M.: The classical complement pathway. Mechanism of activation and regulation. Prog. Allergy, vol. 30, pp. 135–192 (Karger, Basel 1982).

111 Loos, M.; Bitter-Suermann, D.; Dierich, M.: Interaction of the first (C1̄), the second (C2) and the fourth (C4) components of complement with different preparations of bacterial lipopolysaccharides and with lipid A. J. Immun. *112:* 935–940 (1974).

112 Lundh, B.; Hedberg, H.; Laurell, A.-B.: Studies of the third component of complement in synovial fluid from arthritic patients. I. Immunochemical quantitation and relation to total complement. Clin. exp. Immunol. *6:* 407–411 (1970).

113 Lundh, B.; Laurell, A.-B.; Wetterqvist, H.; White, T.; Granerus, G.: A case of hereditary angioneurotic edema successfully treated with ε-aminocaproic acid. Studies on C1

esterase inhibitor, C1 activation, plasminogen level and histamin metabolism. Clin. exp. Immunol. *3:* 733–745 (1968).

114 Mancini, G.; Carbonara, A.O.; Heremans, J.F.: Immunochemical quantitation of antigens by immunodiffusion. Immunochemistry *2:* 235–254 (1965).

115 Manni, A.; Müller-Eberhard, H.J.: The eighth component of human complement (C8). Isolation, characterization and hemolytic efficiency. J. exp. Med. *130:* 1145–1160 (1969).

116 Mathews, K.P.: Management of urticaria and angioedema. J. Allergy clin. Immunol. *66:* 347–357 (1980).

117 Mathews, K.P.: Urticaria and angioedema. J. Allergy clin. Immunol. *72:* 1–14 (1983).

118 Mathews, K.P.; Pan, P.M.; Gardner, N.J.; Hugli, T.E.: Familial carboxypeptidase N deficiency. Ann. intern. Med. *93:* 443–445 (1980).

119 McKay, E.J.; Laurell, A.-B.; Mårtensson, U.; Sjöholm, A.G.: Activation of C1, the first component of complement, the generation of C1r–C1s and $C\bar{1}$ inactivator complexes in normal serum, by heparinaffinity chromatography Mol. Immunol. *18:* 349–357 (1981).

120 Milgrom, H.; Curd, J.G.; Kaplan, R.A.; Müller-Eberhard, H.J.; Vaughan, J.H.: Activation of the fourth component of complement (C4): Assessment by rocket immunoelectrophoresis and correlation with the metabolism of C4. J. Immun. *124:* 2780–2785 (1980).

121 Müller-Eberhard, H.J.; Kunkel, H.G.: Isolation of a thermolabile serum protein which precipitates gammaglobulin aggregates and participates in immune hemolysis. Proc. Soc. exp. Biol. Med. *106:* 291–295 (1961).

122 Müller-Eberhard, H.J.; Schreiber, R.D.: Molecular biology and chemistry of the alternative pathway of complement. Adv. Immunol. *29:* 1–49 (1980).

123 Müller-Eberhard, H.J.; Polley, M.J.; Calcott, M.A.: Formation and functional significance of a molecular complex derived from the second and the fourth component of human complement. J. exp. Med. *125:* 359–380 (1967).

124 Müllertz, S.: Different molecular forms of plasminogen and plasmin produced by urokinase in human plasma and their relations to protease inhibitors and lysis of fibrinogen and fibrin. Biochem. J. *143:* 273–283 (1974).

125 Müllertz, S.; Clemmensen, I.: The primary inhibitor of plasmin in human plasma. Biochem. J. *159:* 545–553 (1976).

126 Natvig, J.B.; Winchester, R.J.: Complement in rheumatoid inflammation. Acta rheum. scand. *15:* 161–168 (1969).

127 Nilsson, I.M.; Andersson, L.; Björkman, S.E.: Epsilon-aminocaproic acid (EACA) as a therapeutic agent. Based on 5 years clinical experience. Acta med. scand., suppl. 448, pp. 1–46 (1966).

128 Nilsson, U.R.; Mandle, R.J., Jr.; McConnell-Mapes, J.A.: Human C3 and C5: Subunit structure and modifications by trypsin and $C\overline{42}$–$C\overline{423}$. J. Immun. *114:* 815–822 (1975).

129 Oberling, F.; Hauptmann, G.; Land, C.M.; Bergerat, J.P.; Mayer, G.; Batzenschlager, A.; Hammann, B.; Gillett, B.: Déficits acquis de l'inhibiteur de la C1 estérase au cours de syndromes lymphoïdes. Nouv. Presse méd. *4:* 2705 (1975).

130 Osler, W.: Hereditary angioneurotic edema. Am. J. med. Sci. *95:* 362–367 (1888).

131 Ohlsson, K.; Balldin, A.; Borgström, A.; Genell, S.: On the role of trypsin and trypsin inhibitors in acute pancreatitis; in McConn, Role of chemical mediators in acute illness and injuries (Raven Press, New York 1982).

132 Patrick, R.A.; Taubman, S.B.; Lepow, I.H.: Cleavage of the fourth component of human complement (C4) by activated C$\bar{1}$s. Immunochemistry *7:* 217–225 (1970).

133 Pensky, J.; Schwick, H.G.: Human serum inhibitor of C1 esterase: identity with neuraminoglycoprotein. Science *163:* 698–699 (1969).

134 Pensky, J.; Levy, L.R.; Lepow, I.H.: Partial purification of a serum inhibitor of C′1 esterase. J. biol. Chem. *236:* 1674–1679 (1961).

135 Pickering, R.J.; Good, R.A.; Kelly, J.R.; Gewurz, H.: Replacement therapy in hereditary angioedema. Successful treatment of two patients with frozen plasma. Lancet *i:* 326–330 (1969).

136 Pitts, J.S.; Donaldson, V.H.; Forristal, J.; Wyatt, R.J.: Remission induced in hereditary angioneurotic edema with an attenuated androgen (danazol): correlation between concentrations of C$\bar{1}$ inhibitor and the fourth and second components of complement. J. Lab. clin. Med. *92:* 501–507 (1978).

137 Podack, E.R.; Biesecker, G.; Kolb, W.P.; Müller-Eberhard, H.J.: The C5b–6 complex: reaction with C7, C8, C9. J. Immun. *121:* 484–490 (1978).

138 Polley, M.J.; Müller-Eberhard, H.J.: The second component of human complement: its isolation, fragmentation by C′1 esterase and incorporation into C′3 convertase. J. exp. Med. *128:* 533–551 (1968).

139 Quastel, M.; Harrison, R.; Cicardi, M.; Alper, C.A.; Rosen, F.S.: Behavior in vivo of normal and dysfunctional C$\bar{1}$ inhibitor in normal subjects and patients with hereditary angioneurotic edema. J. clin. Invest. *71:* 1041–1046 (1983).

140 Ratnoff, O.D.; Lepow, I.H.: Some properties of an esterase derived from preparations of the first component of complement. J. exp. Med. *106:* 327–343 (1957).

141 Ratnoff, O.D.; Naff, G.B.: The conversion of C1s to C1 esterase by plasmin and trypsin. J. exp. Med. *125:* 337–358 (1967).

142 Ratnoff, O.D.; Pensky, J.; Ogston, D.; Naff, G.B.: The inhibition of plasmin, plasma kallikrein, plasma permeability factor and the C1r subcomponent of the first component of complement by C′1 esterase inhibitor. J. exp. Med. *129:* 315–331 (1969).

143 Reid, K.B.M.; Porter, P.R.: The proteolytic activation systems of complement. A. Rev. Biochem. *50:* 433–464 (1981).

144 Rosen, F.S.; Austen, K.F.: Androgen therapy in hereditary angioneurotic edema. New Engl. J. Med. *295:* 1476–1477 (1976).

145 Rosen, F.S.; Charache, P.; Pensky, J.; Donaldson, V.H.: Hereditary angioneurotic edema: two genetic variants. Science *148:* 957–958 (1965).

146 Rosen, F.S.; Alper, C.A.; Pensky, J.; Klemperer, M.R.; Donaldson, V.H.: Genetically determined heterogeneity of the C1 esterase inhibitor in patients with hereditary angioneurotic edema. J. clin. Invest. *50:* 2143–2149 (1971).

147 Rosenfield, S.I.; Staples, P.J.; Leddy, J.P.: Angioedema and hypocomplementemia: unusual feature of lymphoma. J. Allergy clin. Immunol. *55:* 104 (1975).

148 Rother, U.; Till, G.; Vorländer, V.; Hänsch, G.: Complement system; in Dukor, Kallós, Schumberger, West, PAR, pseudo-allergic reactions: cytotoxic and complement mediated reactions, vol. 2, pp. 71–104 (Karger, Basel 1980).

149 Ruddy, S.; Austen, K.F.: C3 inactivator of man. I. Hemolytic measurement by the inactivation of cell-bound C3. J. Immun. *102:* 533–543 (1969).

150 Ruddy, S.; Austen, K.F.: The complement system in rheumatoid arthritis. I. An analysis of complement component activities in rheumatoid synovial fluids. Arthritis Rheum. *13:* 713–723 (1970).

151 Ruddy, S.; Austen, K.F.: Natural control mechanisms of the complement system; in Ingram, Proc. Int. Symp. Biological activities of complement, pp. 13–26 (Karger, Basel 1972).
152 Schapira, M.; Scott, C.F.; Colman, R.W.: Contribution of the plasma protease inhibitors to the activation of kallikrein in plasma. J. clin. Invest. *69:* 462–468 (1982).
153 Schapira, M.; Silver, L.D.; Scott, C.F.; Alvin, H.; Sehmaier, A.H.; Prograis, L.J.; Curd, J.G.; Colman, R.W.: Prekallikrein activation and high molecular-weight kininogen consumption in hereditary angioedema. New Engl. J. Med. *308:* 1050–1053 (1983).
154 Scharfstein, J.; Ferreira, A.; Gigli, I.; Nussenzweig, V.: Human C4 binding protein. I. Isolation and characterization. J. exp. Med. *148:* 207–222 (1978).
155 Scheffer, A.L.; Austen, K.F.; Rosen, F.S.: Tranexamic acid therapy in hereditary angioneurotic edema. New Engl. J. Med. *287:* 452–454 (1972).
156 Scheffer, A.L.; Fearon, D.T.; Austen, K.F.: Clinical and biochemical effects of stanazolol therapy for hereditary angioedema. J. Allergy clin. Immunol. *68:* 181–187 (1981).
157 Schreiber, A.D.; Zweiman, B.; Atkins, P.; Coldwein, F.; Pietra, G.; Atkinson, B.; Abdon, N.I.: Acquired angioedema with lymphoproliferative disorders. Association of $C\bar{1}$ inhibitor deficiency with cellular abnormality. Blood *48:* 567–580 (1976).
158 Schultz, D.R.; Arnold, P.I.: The first component of human complement: on the mechanism of activation by some carbohydrates. J. Immun. *126:* 1994–1998 (1981).
159 Schultze, H.E.; Heide, K.; Haupt, H.: Über ein noch nicht beschriebenes α_1-Glykoprotein des menschlichen Serums. Naturwissenschaften *49:* 133–134 (1962).
160 Siegel, J.; Rent, R.; Gewurz, H.: Interaction of C-reactive protein with the complement system. I. Protamine-induced consumption of complement in acute phase sera. J. exp. Med. *140:* 631–647 (1974).
161 Siegel, J.; Osmand, A.P.; Wilson, M.; Gewurz, H.: Interactions of C-reactive protein with the complement system. II. CRP-mediated consumption of complement by polyactions. J. exp. Med. *142:* 709–721 (1975).
162 Sjöholm, A.G.: Complement components in normal serum and plasma quantitated by electroimmunoassay. Scand. J. Immunol. *4:* 25–30 (1975).
163 Spaulding, W.B.: Methylestosterone therapy for hereditary episodic edema (hereditary angioneurotic edema). Ann. intern. Med. *53:* 739–745 (1960).
164 Sturfelt, G.; Sjöholm, A.G.: Cleavage of C2 in pathological serum and plasma studied by crossed immunoelectrophoresis. Immunobiology *164:* 302 (1983).
165 Sturfelt, G.; Johnson, U.; Sjöholm, A.G.: Sequential studies of complement activation in SLE-indicator value in relation to disease activity. Acta med. scand. (submitted 1984).
166 Sturfelt, G.; Sjöholm, A.G.; Svensson, B.: Complement components, C1 activation and disease activity in SLE. Int. Archs. Allergy appl. Immunol. *70:* 12–18 (1983).
167 Talamo, R.C.; Haber, R.; Austen, K.F.: A radioimmunoassay for bradykinin in plasma and synovial fluid. J. Lab. clin. Med. *74:* 816–827 (1969).
168 Tamura, N.; Nelson, R.A., Jr.: Three naturally occurring inhibitors of components of complement in guinea pig and rabbit serum. J. Immun. *99:* 582–589 (1967).
169 Thompson, R.A.; Lachmann, P.J.: Reactive lysis: the complement mediated lysis of unsensitized cells. I. The characterization of the indicator factor and its identification as C7. J. exp. Med. *131:* 629–657 (1970).
170 Tomasi, T.B.; Hauptmann, S.P.: The binding of α_1-antitrypsin to human IgA. J. Immun. *112:* 2274–2277 (1974).
171 Truedsson, L.; Sjöholm, A.G.; Laurell, A.-B.: Screening for the classical and alternative

pathways of complement by hemolysis in gel. Acta pathol. microbiol. scand., C, Immunol. *89:* 161–164 (1981).

172 Westaby, D.; Ogle, S.J.; Paradinas, F.J.; Randell, J.B.; Murray-Lyon, I.M.: Liver damage from long-term methyltestosterone. Lancet *ii* 261–263 (1977).

173 Willms, K.; Rosen, F.S.; Donaldson, V.H.: Observations on the ultrastructure of lesions induced in humans and guinea pig skin by C1 esterase and polypeptide from hereditary angioneurotic edema (HANE) plasma. Clin. Immunol. Immunopathol. *4:* 174–188 (1975).

174 Ziccardi, R.J.: Activation of the early components of the classical pathway under physiological conditions. J. Immun. *126:* 1769–1773 (1981).

175 Ziccardi, R.J.: The first component of complement, C1: Activation and control. Springer Semin. Immunopathol. *6:* 213–230 (1983).

176 Ziccardi, R.J.; Cooper, N.R.: Physicochemical and functional characterization of C1r subunit of the first complement component. J. Immun. *116:* 496–503 (1976).

177 Ziccardi, R.J.; Cooper, N.R.: Activation of C1r by proteolytic cleavage. J. Immun. *116:* 504–509 (1976).

178 Ziccardi, R.J.; Cooper, N.R.: Modulation of the antigenicity of C$\bar{1}$r and C$\bar{1}$s by C$\bar{1}$ inactivator. J. Immun. *121:* 2148–2152 (1978).

179 Ziccardi, R.J.; Cooper, N.R.: Active dissassembly of the first complement component, C$\bar{1}$, by C$\bar{1}$ inactivator. J. Immun. *123:* 788–792 (1979).

180 Ziccardi, R.J.; Cooper, N.R.: Development of an immunochemical test to assess C$\bar{1}$ inactivator function in human serum and its use for diagnosis of hereditary angioneurotic edema. Clin. Immunol. Immunopathol. *15:* 465–471 (1980).

A.-B. Laurell, MD, Department of Medical Microbiology,
Sölvegatan 23, S-223 62 Lund (Sweden)

PAR. Pseudo-Allergic Reactions. Involvement of Drugs and Chemicals, vol. 4, pp. 47–58 (Karger, Basel 1985)

Idiopathic and Exercise-Induced 'Anaphylaxis'[1]

Lee Sonin, Roy Patterson

Section of Allergy-Immunology, Department of Medicine, Northwestern University Medical School, Chicago, Ill., USA

Introduction

Three syndromes, idiopathic anaphylaxis (IA), exercise-induced anaphylaxis (EA), and food-dependent exercise-induced anaphylaxis (FEA) are pseudo-allergic reactions. Their symptoms mimic immediate antigen-mediated systemic reactions but etiologic antigens have not been found. As these reactions are life-threatening, it is essential that the physician is aware of them. A clinical summary with a discussion of each of these syndromes is presented in this review.

Idiopathic Anaphylaxis

IA [1–4] is a life-threatening systemic reaction of unknown etiology manifested by urticaria or angioedema associated with upper airway obstruction, bronchospasm, hypotension or syncope, and gastrointestinal symptoms. All symptoms may not be present in each patient or at each recurrence. These patients do not have anaphylaxis from known IgE-mediated causes such as foods, drugs or Hymenoptera stings or from non-IgE-mediated pseudo-allergic causes such as iodinated radiographic contrast media [5] or exercise [6].

Once a diagnosis of IA is suspected, repeated efforts should be made to identify any known causes of anaphylaxis. Patients should be instructed

[1] Supported by USPHS grant AI 11403 and the Ernest S. Bazley Grant.

to keep food diaries for evaluation by their physicians. Systemic illness that might mimic anaphylaxis, such as hereditary angioneurotic edema, systemic mastocytosis, carcinoid syndrome, vasculitis or collagen vascular disease, must also be considered. Factitious disease is always a consideration to be excluded [7].

We have studied a group of 50 patients with IA [4]. All patients had urticaria or angioedema. 66% of the patients had associated gastrointestinal symptoms, bronchospasm, hypotension or syncope. The other 34% of the patients had life-threatening upper airway obstruction without the other associated symptoms. Table I shows the symptoms in these patients. In addition to repeated histories and physical examinations, laboratory studies that may be helpful are listed in table II. Some routine laboratory examinations are recommended, as are selected studies in patients whose symptoms are suggestive of one of the systemic diseases previously listed.

6 of 26 patients tested had abnormal erythrocyte sedimentation rates, but 1 of these patients also had a preleukemic syndrome. 7 of 32 patients had abnormal CH_{50} values. 1 patient had a low C4 value with normal C1 esterase inhibitor levels. Food skin tests were negative in 21 patients, and 25 of 28 patients had positive cutaneous tests to common inhalant antigens. None of these patients had celery anaphylaxis.

In the 18 patients reported by *Lieberman and Taylor* [2], the results of most laboratory examinations were unremarkable. Erythrocyte sedimentation rates were not done. Complement levels were normal in 13 patients tested, except for 1 patient with a low C4 during an attack which subsequently returned to normal, and then remained normal during the next attack. All patients had negative food skin tests and none of 3 patients tested were atopic.

One patient with IA reported by *Greenberger* [8], was found to have an elevated serum IgE of 23,136 ng/ml. This patient had life-threatening episodes of IA associated with orthostatic hypotension, small bowel obstruction and ischemic electrocardiographic changes. Three episodes were preceded by substantial increases in the total serum IgE which subsequently returned to a baseline value. Extensive evaluations including laparotomy did not reveal an etiology in this patient. A similar serologic pattern has not been discovered in other patients with IA.

Lieberman and Taylor [2] felt that prophylactic medication was of no benefit to their patients. Antihistaminic and sympathomimetic medications, and prednisone in 2 patients were tried. For acute reactions, epinephrine injection by the physician or self-administration was effective.

Table I. Symptoms in 50 patients with IA

Symptom	Incidence %
Angioedema	96
Upper airway obstruction	76
Urticaria	72
Bronchospasm	48
Gastrointestinal	32
Syncope or hypotension	28
Dizziness	8
Nasal symptoms	6

From *Sonin* et al. [4] with permission.

Table II. Laboratory examinations in IA

Routine studies
Complete blood count
Differential leukocyte count
Urinalysis
Erythrocyte sedimentation rate
Studies to be considered for selected patients
Blood chemistries
C3 C4 CH_{50}
$C\bar{1}$ esterase inhibitor levels
5-Hydroxyindoleacetic acid
Bone marrow aspiration
Cutaneous food testing by the prick method

Our treatment experience [1, 3, 4] is summarized in table III. For infrequent reactions, patients are instructed to administer 0.3 cm^3 of 1:1,000 epinephrine subcutaneously and to take an oral dosage of 40 mg of prednisone and an antihistamine immediately. Patients then proceed to the emergency room or call our emergency number for further advice.

In contrast to *Lieberman and Taylor* [2], we have found that prophylactic medication is helpful in preventing frequently recurring reactions [1, 3, 4]. Patients with frequent reactions proceed as above for an acute reaction. To stabilize their condition, regular dose antihistamines are admi-

Table III. Treatment of IA

Acute reaction
Self-injection of 0.3 cm^3 1:1,000 epinephrine subcutaneously
Oral dose of 40 mg prednisone and an antihistamine
Call emergency number or proceed to emergency room for further treatment
Patient with infrequent reactions
Treatment as in 'Acute reaction'
Patient with frequent reactions
Emergency therapy as in 'Acute reaction'
Trial of regular dose of antihistamines
For severe reactions or reactions uncontrolled by antihistamines
40 mg prednisone daily (higher if necessary) until symptoms are controlled
Institute alternate-day prednisone with a very slow decrease once symptoms are controlled
Continuous antihistamines

nistered. For severe reactions or for patients not controlled on antihistamines alone, 40 mg of daily prednisone is added. Once patients are stabilized, alternate-day prednisone is initiated and corticosteroids are slowly tapered down.

A patient may require a maintenance dosage of anthistamines or alternate-day prednisone to prevent further episodes of idiopathic anaphylaxis. Patients taking corticosteroids to prevent episodes of IA require much lower doses of alternate-day prednisone that the daily doses needed to establish control of symptoms. Patients not in remission continue to have urticaria or angioedema controlled by medication.

Of 50 patients [4], 7 are in remission totalling 20 patient years. Remission is defined as absence of symptoms for 1 year off all prophylactic medication. 21 patients require regular medication, with 17 on alternate-day prednisone. 14 patients require intermittent medication for infrequent reactions. Medication was not helpful in 2 patients, but 1 refused a trial of prednisone and the other was lost to follow-up. 7 patients were lost to follow-up. No anaphylactic deaths occurred during 292 patient years of symptoms and 161 patient years of follow-up.

Lieberman and Taylor [2] followed up 10 of their patients. There were no deaths, and 5 of the patients were in remission. The other patients continued to experience attacks of idiopathic anaphylaxis.

The pathogenesis of IA is unknown. Most patients are atopic [4]. 3 patients had elevated serum histamine levels [1, 2] and 2 patients had elevated urine histamine levels [9] during attacks of IA. These results prompted us to look for a cellular mechanism. These patients might have basophils and mast cells that exhibit enhanced histamine release. A basophil-rich leukocyte fraction was separated from the blood of 6 non-atopic control subjects and 7 patients with IA. Spontaneous histamine release and histamine release induced by anti-human IgE was measured [unpublished data]. There was no significant difference in spontaneous or anti-IgE-induced histamine release between the two groups.

Some of our patients had abnormal erythrocyte sedimentation rates and complement values. The significance of this is unknown. During an episode of IA, a patient might develop complement pathway activation with generation of anaphylatoxins and subsequent mediator release causing the syndrome. There was no difference in the nature or severity of IA in patients with abnormal laboratory values [4].

Patients and referring physicians often incriminate foods or food additives as the cause of a patient's symptoms. A food-precipitating anaphylaxis is usually known to the patient but, in some of our patients after extensive review of their food diaries, a specific food has been identified [1, 10, 11]. A food or additive is not suspected in the great majority of our patients because reactions have occurred more than 4 h after ingestion.

In searching for an etiologic cause of these episodes, we have investigated one of the sulphiting agents, sodium metabisulphite. The sulphite salts and sulphur dioxide are a group of compounds generally regarded as safe for use in foods not containing thiamine by the US Food and Drug Administration. These compounds are used for their antimicrobial actions and preservative effects on foods. They are often used in beers, wines, fresh and dehydrated fruits and vegetables, and shellfish. They are most commonly used by caterers or restaurants in salads, potatoes and avocado dips. Outside the United States, sulphite salts are used more commonly in fresh meats, meat products and fish [12]. A restaurant meal may contain up to 100 mg of these sulphite salts [13]. Sulphiting agents have also been used as preservatives in some parenteral medications [14, 15].

It has been suggested by some authors that sulphiting agents are the cause of anaphylactoid reactions in some patients. Bronchospasm is the major symptom in these reports [13–15]. In one case report [16], urticaria and angioedema were the prominent symptoms and, in 2 patients presented [17], the systemic symptoms experienced by the patients did not appear to be allergic or anaphylactoid in nature.

We challenged 12 IA patients with one of the sulphiting agents, sodium metabisulphite. 8 patients had symptoms associated with restaurant meals, possibly due to sulphiting agents. The other 4 were challenged to determine if sulphites might be a hidden cause. Patients received oral doses of 1, 5, 10, 25, 50, 100, 200 mg for a total dosage of 391 mg, which is about 4 times more than would be ingested in a heavily sulphited restaurant meal. Prick cutaneous tests were negative in all patients. No symptoms suggestive of IA or immediate hypersensitivity occurred during sodium metabisulphite test dosing in the 12 patients. Our conclusion was that sulphiting agents are not the cause of IA in our 12 patients tested. One of our IA patients also received an oral tartrazine challenge (81 mg total dose) with no reaction.

Food additives may be incriminated as the cause of anaphylactoid or other reactions. Tartrazine was initially felt to be a common precipitant of allergic reactions, but in clinical practice tartrazine sensitivity appears to be very rare. The physician must keep an open mind in searching for etiologic causes of allergic or pseudo-allergic reactions, but when investigating food additives or other compounds, the physician needs to remain objective and to free himself from any preconceived notions.

With the program outlined in table III, no anaphylactic deaths have occurred, and patients are able to resume and maintain a productive lifestyle.

Exercise-Induced Anaphylaxis and Food-Dependent Exercise-Induced Anaphylaxis

Anaphylaxis has been recognized as a manifestation of physical allergy. Patients with cold-induced urticaria can become hypotensive with exposure of their bodies to the cold [18, 19] and a rare patient with cholinergic urticaria developed hypotension with exercise [20]. EA [6, 21, 22] is a newly recognized syndrome where a patient develops exercise-induced symptoms of generalized pruritus, urticaria or angioedema, hypotension, upper airway obstruction, gastrointestinal symptoms, headache, or wheezing [6]. All of these patients have exercise-induced urticaria or angioedema in addition to their other anaphylactic symptoms. These symptoms are shown in table IV. EA is another life-threatening exercise-related

Table IV. Symptoms in 16 patients with EA

Symptoms	Incidence %
Urticaria or angioedema	100
Urticaria	94
Collapse	75
Choking	63
Angioedema	56
Bronchospasm	44
Gastrointestinal symptoms	31
Headache	25
Rhinitis	13

From *Sheffer and Austin* [6].

syndrome in addition to syncope [23] and collapse with myocardial infarction [24].

Patients developed symptoms with jogging, sprinting, tennis, basketball, dancing, squash and marching. They develop prodromal symptoms of pruritus, erythema, or urticarial lesions, and further progression of the reaction may be aborted if the patient stops exercise at this point. There is no regular consistency to this syndrome. A degree of physical exertion may provoke anaphylaxis at one time but not at another with similar degree of exercise [6, 22].

Extensive histories were taken to eliminate other known causes of anaphylaxis. Routine hematology studies, blood chemistries, levels of C3 and C4, total hemolytic complement (CH_{50}) and quantitative immunoglobulins were normal [6]. *Sheffer and Austen* [6] had 6 of 16 patients and *Songsiridej and Busse* [22] had 5 of 7 patients with EA that were atopic. Interestingly, 2 of 16 patients described also had cold-induced urticaria [6].

Patients with EA are treated acutely, as would any other patient with anaphylaxis. Epinephrine injection is effective [6, 22]. Antihistamines are helpful and if necessary intravenous fluids and vasoactive drugs may be administered. For a life-threatening reaction, we recommend a short course of corticosteroids with careful monitoring of the patients' condition.

All patients should be instructed in the self-administration of epinephrine. For life-threatening reactions, we recommend that the patients limit their exercise program, due to the unpredictable nature of this syndrome. Those patients who insist on continuing their exercise program are instructed to participate with someone who understands their syndrome and is able to administer epinephrine. Prevention of severe reactions may occur if the patient stops his exertion immediately at the onset of any prodromal symptoms; continuation of exercise results in a more severe attack [6, 22]. We do not recommend exercise until prodromal symptoms occur because, if the reaction continued to progress after exertion is stopped, the potential of a death exists. *Sheffer and Austen* [6] felt that antihistamine drugs administered on a regular basis or before exercise were helpful but not completely effective in preventing attacks.

Sheffer et al. [21] performed exercise challenges on 7 patients with EA. Patients wearing occlusive suits were instructed to run on a treadmill. 4 of 7 patients had abnormal exercise tests. Each of these patients developed cutaneous pruritus and erythema without urticaria. 2 subjects developed angioedema, 1 with upper respiratory obstruction and cough requiring epinephrine injection. Pulmonary function testing showed no significant change.

Baseline and exercise histamine levels were measured. Whole blood histamine increased with exercise in asthmatics and control patients due to a rise in the basophil count, but there was no increase in the plasma histamine measured in venous blood samples [30]. The patients who had a clinical response to exercise challenge had a higher peak exercise serum histamine level than did those patients who did not have a response to exercise challenge [21].

Some patients with cholinergic urticaria have exercise-induced hypotension, a syndrome similar to EA. *Kaplan* et al. [20] described 2 EA patients with punctate lesions typical of cholinergic urticaria [25]. One of these patients had urticarial lesions associated with warm showers, but the other patient only had exercise-induced symptoms. Both patients had an exercise challenge on a bicycle ergometer. Both patients also developed cholinergic urticarial lesions and angioedema and 1 patient developed hypotension. Plasma histamine levels were elevated in both patients. Pulmonary function tests showed no change with exercise.

Lewis et al. [26] performed exercise challenges in patients with exercise-induced anaphylactoid symptoms. During free running 2 of their patients developed EA with hypotension and elevated plasma histamine, requiring epinephrine injection for control of their symptoms. The urticarial lesions were giant urticaria in 1 patient and of the cholinergic type in the other. The patient with cholinergic urticaria also had cold-induced urticaria.

Mediator release has been studied in patients with cholinergic urticaria. 2 patients [19] with typical cholinergic urticaria developed increased plasma histamine levels during and after strenuous exercise. Another patient tested by the same authors had elevated baseline and exercise serotonin levels, but normal levels of histamine. Patients with cholinergic urticaria and exercise-induced bronchospasm have been described [27–29]. One of these patients also had dermographism [27].

Soter et al. [29] had 7 patients with cholinergic urticaria exercise by running in place on a treadmill wearing a plastic occlusive suit to raise their core body temperature. All patients developed pinpoint urticaria, and wheezing was detected by auscultation in 4 of 7 patients. Pulmonary function testing showed significant falls in FEV_1, MMF, and SGaw, with an increase in the residual volume. Serum taken during exercise showed increased levels of histamine and an augmentation of eosinophil and neutrophil chemotactic activities.

These studies show that mediators may be released during exercise challenge in patients with EA and cholinergic urticaria. *Sheffer* et al. [21] felt that there are 3 separate types of exercise-induced physical allergy. Each type has been shown to have elevated serum histamine levels during exercise challenge. The first type is typical cholinergic urticaria which is also precipitated by heat and stress. This type may be associated with bronchospasm, but not hypotension or syncope. Secondly, there is EA where the urticarial lesions are of the conventional type. The third type is called variant syndrome because its clinical expression is a blending of the first two. The urticarial lesions are punctate, but these patients also develop hypotension or syncope. 2 of the 16 patients originally described by *Sheffer and Austen* [6] had this syndrome.

2 families have been reported in abstracts [31, 32] where 1 individual had EA with siblings who had exercise-induced urticaria or angioedema, but no anaphylactic symptoms.

A subset of EA patients has FEA [33–35]. *Sheffer* et al. [6] noted that 3 of their 16 patients had more severe episodes of EA when their exertion was postprandial, in contrast to this group of patients where anaphylaxis does not occur unless both food ingestion and physical exertion occur together. It is important to note that patients with FEA develop reactions with food ingestion plus exercise. This is not food allergy plus exercise.

Maulitz et al. [33] described a 31-year-old male long-distance runner who had 3 post-exercise episodes of urticaria and upper airway closure requiring epinephrine and antihistamines. The first episode was preceeded by shrimp ingestion 5 h before and the other episodes were preceeded by smoked oyster ingestion 20 and 24 h beforehand. No reactions occurred with exercise or shellfish ingestion alone. The patient had positive prick tests to oysters and shrimp.

Kidd et al. [34] described 4 patients with FEA. 2 patients developed anaphylaxis when they exercised within 2 h after celery ingestion, and 1 patient when celery was ingested within 2 h following exercise. These patients were prick-test positive to celery. A 4th patient developed anaphylaxis upon exertion within 2 h after food ingestion. 3 of the 4 patients had documented hypotension requiring epinephrine injection and antihistamines to reverse the reaction. The patients with FEA associated with celery had allergic rhinitis. Patients prevented further episodes of FEA by avoiding exercise temporarily related to food or celery ingestion.

Novey et al. [35] reported on a 41-year-old male who had multiple episodes of anaphylaxis when he exercised within 2 h of a meal. This patient had severe reactions with syncopal episodes. 3 exercise challenges were performed on a bicycle ergometer; fasting with heat-dissipating clothing, fasting with a plastic occlusive suit, and postprandially with heat-dissipating clothing. During the first 2 studies in the fasting state, the patient developed a few small urticarial lesions. In the postprandial test, the patient developed mild angioedema of the eyes and hypotension. Laboratory studies showed no significant changes in pulmonary function testing or plasma histamine levels, or evidence of complement activation.

Each patient with FEA developed their systemic reactions only with the association of nonspecific or specific food ingestion and exercise. Exercise or food ingestion alone would not precipitate the syndrome clinically, except for 1 patient who developed a few urticarial lesions during exercise challenge while fasting [35]. Only 6 patients have been reported with the FEA syndrome. In 2 patients unusual circumstances exist. Immediate hypersensitivity reactions did not occur 24 h after food ingestion, but they occurred in the patient with shellfish-associated FEA [33]. The patient with postprandial FEA did develop urticarial lesions during exercise challenge in a fasting state [35] which suggests that he might have EA worse after food ingestion, similar to some of the other patients with EA previously described [6]. FEA is an unusual syndrome and it will be important to see whether other patients are described in the future with this syndrome to extend the understanding of this problem.

References

1 Bacal, E.; Patterson, R.; Zeiss, C.R.: Evaluation of severe (anaphylactic) reactions. Clin. Allergy *8:* 295–304 (1978).
2 Lieberman, P.; Taylor, W.W.: Recurrent idiopathic anaphylaxis. Archs intern. Med. *139:* 1032–1034 (1979).
3 Sale, S.R.; Greenberger, P.A.; Patterson, R.: Idiopathic anaphylactoid reactions. J. Am. med. Ass. *246:* 2336–2339 (1981).
4 Sonin, L.; Grammer, L.G.; Greenberger, P.A.; Patterson, R.: Idiopathic anaphylaxis: a clinical summary. Ann. intern. Med. *99:* 634–635 (1983).
5 Austen, K.F.: Systemic anaphylaxis in man. J. Am. med. Ass. *192:* 108–110 (1965).
6 Sheffer, A.L.; Austen, K.F.: Exercise-induced anaphylaxis. J. Allergy clin. Immunol. *66:* 106–111 (1980).
7 Patterson, R.; Schatz, M.; Horton, M.: Munchausen's stridor: non-organic laryngeal obstruction. Clin. Allergy *4:* 307–310 (1974).
8 Greenberger, P.A.: A case of life-threatening idiopathic anaphylactoid reactions associated with hyperimmunoglobulinemia E. Am. J. Med. (in press).
9 Myers, G.; Donlon, M.; Kaliner, M.: Measurement of urinary histamine: Development of methodology and normal values. J. Allergy clin. Immunol. *67:* 305–311 (1981).
10 Golbert, T.M.; Patterson, R.; Pruzansky, J.: Systemic allergic reactions to ingested allergens. J. Allergy clin. Immunol. *44:* 96–107 (1969).
11 Patterson, R.; Schatz, M.: Factitious allergic emergencies: anaphylaxis and laryngeal edema. J. Allergy clin. Immunol. *56:* 152–159 (1975).
12 Furia, T.E.: Handbook of food additives, pp. 142–147 (CRC Press, Cleveland 1972).
13 Stevenson, D.D.; Simon, R.A.: Sensitivity to ingested metabisulfites in asthmatic subjects. J. Allergy clin. Immunol. *68:* 26–32 (1981).
14 Baker, G.J.; Collett, P.; Allen, D.H.: Bronchospasm induced by metabisulfite-containing foods and drugs. Med. J. Aust. *2:* 614–616 (1981).
15 Twarog, F.J.; Leung, D.Y.: Anaphylaxis to a component of isoethanine (sodium bisulfite). J. Am. med. Ass. *248:* 2030–2031 (1982).
16 Prenner, B.M.; Stevens, J.J.: Anaphylaxis after ingestion of sodium bisulfite. Ann. Allergy *37:* 180–182 (1976).
17 Schwartz, H.J.: Sensitivity to ingested metabisulfite: variations in clinical presentation. J. Allergy clin. Immunol. *71:* 487–489 (1983).
18 Horton, B.T.; Brown, G.E.; Roth, G.M.: Hypersensitivities to cold with local and systemic manifestations of a histamine-like character: Its amendability to treatment. J. Am. med. Ass. *107:* 1263–1269 (1936).
19 Kaplan, A.P.; Gray, L.; Shaff, R.E.; Horakova, Z.; Beaven, M.A.: In vivo studies of mediator release in cold urticaria and cholinergic urticaria. J. Allergy clin. Immunol. *55:* 394–402 (1975).
20 Kaplan, A.P.; Natbony, S.F.; Tawil, A.P.; Fruchter, L.; Foster, M.: Exercise-induced anaphylaxis as a manifestation of cholergic urticaria. J. Allergy clin. Immunol. *68:* 319–324 (1981).
21 Sheffer, A.L.; Soter, N.A.; McFadden, E.R., Jr.; Auster, K.F.: Exercise-induced anaphylaxis: a distince force of physical allergy. J. Allergy clin. Immunol. *71:* 311–316 (1983).

22 Songsiridej, V.; Busse, W.W.: Exercise-induced anaphylaxis. Clin. Allergy *13:* 317–321 (1983).

23 Tsutsumi, E.; Hara, H.: Syncope after running. Br. med. J. *ii:* 1480 (1979).

24 Green, L.H.; Cohen, S.I.; Kurland, G.: Fatal myocardial infarction in marathon racing. Ann. intern. Med. *84:* 704–706 (1976).

25 Great, R.T.; Pearson, R.S.B.; Comean, W.J.: Observation on urticaria provoked by emotion, by exercise, and by warming of the body. Clin. Sci. *2:* 253–272 (1936).

26 Lewis, J.; Lieberman, P.; Treadwell, G.; Erffmeyer, J.: Exercise-induced urticaria, angioedema, and anaphylactoid episodes. J. Allergy clin. Immunol. *68:* 432–437 (1981).

27 Mathews, K.P.; Pan, P.M.: Postexercise hyperhistaminemia, dermographia, and wheezing. Ann. intern. Med. *72:* 241–249 (1970).

28 Blumberg, M.Z.: Cholinergic urticaria and asthma: a case report. Ann. Allergy *41:* 99–100 (1978).

29 Soter, N.A.; Wasserman, S.I.; Austen, K.F.; McFadden, E.R., Jr.: Release of mast-cell mediators and alternations in lung function in patients with cholinergic urticaria. New Engl. J. Med. *302:* 604–608 (1980).

30 Harris, M.G.; Burge, P.S.; O'Brien, L.; Cromwell, O.; Pepys, J.: Blood histamine levels after exercise testing. Clin. Allergy *9:* 437–441 (1979).

31 Grant, J.A.; Schmalstieg, F.; Fine, D.P.; Lord, R.: Familial exercise-induced anaphylaxis (Abstract). J. Allergy clin. Immunol. *69:* 103 (1982).

32 Longley, S.; Scornik, J.; Panush, R.; Katz, P.: Familial exercise-induced anaphylaxis (Abstract). J. Allergy clin. Immunol. *69:* 103 (1982).

33 Maulitz, R.M.; Pratt, D.S.; Schocket, A.L.: Exercise-induced anaphylactic reaction to shellfish. J. Allergy clin. Immunol. *63:* 433–434 (1979).

34 Kidd, J.M., III; Cohen, S.H.; Sosman, A.J.; Fink, N.J.: Food-dependent exercise-induced anaphylaxis. J. Allergy clin. Immunol. *71:* 407–411 (1983).

35 Novey, H.S.; Fairshter, R.D.; Salness, K.; Simon, R.A.; Curd, J.G.: Postprandial exercise-induced anaphylaxis. J. Allergy clin. Immunol. *71:* 498–504 (1983).

R. Patterson, MD, 303 East Chicago Avenue, Chicago, IL 60611 (USA)

PAR. Pseudo-Allergic Reactions. Involvement of Drugs and Chemicals, vol. 4, pp. 59–105 (Karger, Basel 1985)

Allergomimetic Reactions to Food and Pseudo-Food-Allergy

David J. Pearson, Keith J.B. Rix

University of Manchester and University of Leeds, England

Introduction

Reactions to food as a counterpart to experimental anaphylaxis in animals were recognized by 1908 [74]. It soon became apparent that not all food hypersensitivity is due to what would now be considered IgE-mediated allergy. It is now clear not only that adverse reactions to foods can be produced by a variety of psychological and physical mechanisms, but also that individual types of reaction can be responsible for differing clinical syndromes.

There was a vogue in the 1920s and 1930s for incriminating food allergy in virtually all hitherto unexplained phenomena [49, 52, 137, 162, 166]. A reaction to some of the more uncritical and overenthusiastic of these claims, which were often based on anecdotal evidence and misunderstanding of the limitations of available diagnostic techniques, led to a widespread disenchantment with the subject which inhibited its scientific study for many years. Recent advances in the understanding of hypersensitivity responses in general have produced a renewed interest in food-induced reactions. Unfortunately this has been associated with renewed suggestions, based on questionable evidence, that food allergy is a common cause of a wide range of non-atopic conditions [96, 128]. If we are to avoid the errors of the past, it is crucial that we maintain a critical, objective and scientific attitude, applying strict criteria to both terminology and diagnosis.

Classification of Adverse Reactions to Food

Clear definitions of terminology promote clarity of thinking and allow accurate communication. In classical immunological usage *allergy*

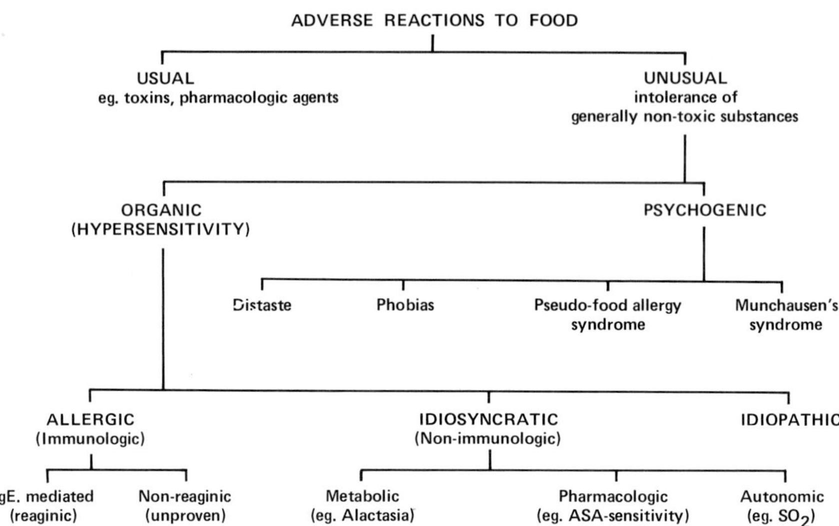

Fig. 1. Schematic representation of reactions to foods.

describes any form of specific altered reactivity secondary to previous exposure [31]. Many patients equate the term with any negative reaction and some professional groups apply it to all idiosyncratic or acquired adverse reactions [124]. This leads to several problems: it obscures the heterogeneity of reactions and therefore obstructs their elucidation; although the occurrence of one type of response in an individual does not necessarily predispose to the production of another, the opposite may be assumed by describing both as 'allergy'; it may also lead to the misapplication of diagnostic techniques suitable for one type of sensitivity but not another.

Figure 1 shows our classification of adverse reactions to foods. First there are those *usual* reactions which occur in virtually all individuals ingesting a sufficient quantity of a particular substance. These would include responses to chemical and bacterial toxins; effects of naturally occurring pharmacological agents (e.g. in coffee, tea, and alcoholic beverages, etc.); and alterations in gastrointestinal function with fibre intake. *Unusual reactions* occur in some individuals who react to substances which are eaten without ill-effect by most of the population. We subdivide this *intolerance* into *psychogenic* and *organic* (hypersensitivity).

Since the commonest cause of failing to tolerate specific foods may be psychological [90], it seems misleading to imply an organic aetiology by the use of intolerance. However, an inclusive term is required to describe all organic 'unusual' reactions. We believe there is historical precedence for using hypersensitivity in this context. Consequently, we define *hypersensitivity* as: 'An organic host-damaging reaction which is qualitatively different from, or quantitatively greater than, the effects that the same dose of that substance would have on the generality of the population'. This definition has no implications as to the type of organic process involved. It includes enhanced susceptibility to the usual effects of pharmacological and toxic agents, as well as allergic and pseudo-allergic reactions. It does suffer from the shortcoming that, as discussed in volume 1 of this series, hypersensitivity can be taken to imply a purely quantitative difference in reactivity. However, in allergic and allergomimetic reactions, in which particular substances have an apparently qualitatively different effect, the *hypersensitivity* can be conceived as being in the release/generation of usual endogenous mediators.

We would prefer *allergic food hypersensitivity* as a more explicit definition of immunologically-mediated adverse reactions to food, but we are prepared to apply *food allergy* to this state, since the term has such wide usage in this context. Although particular allergies occur in a restricted proportion of the population, we retain *idiosyncrasy* for non-immunological reactions, which are peculiar to only certain individuals, and which are related to the metabolic or pharmacological properties of the inciting substance. Examples covered by the last would include aspirin intolerance and the response to milk in genetically alactasic patients.

In discussing reactions which may be confused with true food allergy we must also make some further distinctions. First, although IgE-mediated hypersensitivity is the only immunological mechanism whose role has been demonstrated convincingly, other forms of food allergy probably exist (e.g. in coeliac disease). However, since they are so poorly understood at the present time, they will not be discussed further here. Secondly, we must distinguish between non-immunological organic processes which resemble known allergic reactions; and states which are attributed to food allergy, in the absence of evidence for any form of organic sensitivity. In this chapter we shall use *anaphylactoid* to describe allergomimetic organic reactions which resemble IgE-mediated hypersensitivity (i.e. type 1 PAR).

We shall reserve *pseudo-food allergy* for the mistaken belief in food allergy as the cause of any symptoms, whether or not these resemble those of recognized allergic disease.

Anaphylactoid Reactions to Foods

Genuine IgE-mediated food allergy may cause anaphylactic shock, urticaria, asthma, rhinitis, eczema, vomiting, abdominal pain and diarrhoea, and in a proportion of patients abdominal symptoms predominate [91]. Therefore, virtually any diarrhoeal process could be considered as anaphylactoid. However, since space prevents a comprehensive review of the role of foods in the production of diarrhoea, we shall merely consider briefly the most important responses to ingested substances which may reproduce the other major manifestations of atopy. The most frequent of these are sensitivity to compounds which may cross-react with aspirin; and bronchospastic responses to sulphur dioxide and related food preservatives.

Intolerance to Aspirin, Azo Dyes and Benzoate Food Preservatives

Intolerance to aspirin (acetylsalicylic acid, ASA) was reviewed in the first volume of this series [144]. Therefore, we shall discuss only those aspects of this syndrome which are of particular relevance to food-related anaphylactoid reactions. Reactions to ASA are only one aspect of a syndrome in which hypersensitivity to any of a group of substances can occur. Adverse reactions to more than 80 other unrelated substances have been reported in ASA-intolerant patients [144]. Most individuals with this syndrome will react to only a limited number of these and sensitivity to other members of the group can occur in the absence of intolerance to ASA itself [105, 144]. ASA-sensitive patients may react to certain foods containing natural cross-reacting substances, as well as to foods and medicines containing artificial azo colouring and benzoate preservative agents [25, 40, 94, 105, 138, 151] (table I).

Adverse reactions in the ASA-intolerance syndrome vary in severity from simple urticaria, through rhinitis, asthma and angioedema, to an immediate shocked state resembling anaphylaxis. There is no evidence to incriminate a specific immune process in most cases. Although the syndrome may not be expressed until later life, it is likely that it is a genetically determined, idiosyncratic response which is inherited independently

Table I. Possible food reactions in ASA intolerance syndrome

Additives	Natural products
Dyes	Peas
Amaranth	Liquorice
Erythrosine	Bananas
Ponceau 4R	Rhubarb
Sunset yellow	Berries
Tartrazine	Apples
	Grapes
Preservatives	Ciders
Sodium benzoate	Wines
4-Hydroxybenzoic acid esters	Beers

from atopy [144]. Patients developing asthma after ASA ingestion have the same incidence of inhalant sensitivities as does the general asthmatic population [102], whereas it is notable that patients with chronic urticaria without asthma, are predominantly non-atopic [26].

Intolerance to ASA and/or other cross-reacting substances is common in patients presenting with either asthma [122, 151, 153, 165] or chronic urticaria [26, 40, 105]. Many are unaware of their sensitivity [102, 122]. Based on oral challenge studies, the prevalence of ASA intolerance in chronic asthma appears to be between 12 and 28%. Estimates of the frequency of these intolerances in chronic urticaria vary more markedly (between 22 and 67%), but suggest a considerably higher frequency in this population [144].

Azo dyes such as tartrazine are contained in many pills, capsules and elixirs and are also used widely in the food-manufacturing industry to impart red or yellow colouration, or to maintain a 'fresh' appearance in pre-packed meats. They are common in cordials and other drinks (particularly orangeades and squashes); preserved and smoked meats and fishes (e.g. smoked and unsmoked pork products, haddock, etc.); coloured cheeses and many 'convenience foods'. Sodium benzoate and other benzoic acid derivatives are used as food preservatives. They are found commonly in products sold for later cooking (e.g. some white flours, sausages, minced meats, etc.), as well as pre-prepared foods.

The high frequency with which artificial dyes and preservatives occur in the western diet can lead to chronic unremitting symptoms and make recognition of the sensitivity difficult. In addition, their presence can lead to natural foods being blamed mistakenly for acute reactions. The latter is a problem in improperly performed food exclusion-reintroduction protocols, particularly when these are self-administered. However, patients can react to certain unadulterated foods some of which are considered to contain natural salicylates or benzoates [105]. Diagnosis of ASA intolerance is confirmed by oral provocation. However, initial doses need to be small and incremental doses given at not more than 2- to 3-hour intervals. We have observed 30% falls in FEV_1 with as little as 1 mg of ASA. Although some published series suggest that reactions to ASA abate within 4 h [37], we have seen the FEV_1 continue to fall for more than 5 h and not return to baseline until after 24 h. Investigation of dye and preservative intolerance is complicated by the number of potential agents to be tested in provocation studies and by the fact that patients often react to a limited number of these. However, a therapeutic trial of a diet excluding all these substances should indicate the potential value of further investigations.

The optimum treatment of this syndrome is uncertain. Although there are numerous reports that suitable dietary avoidance is effective in the control of chronic urticaria [40, 63, 135], its proper role in asthma is uncertain. It seems obvious that patients with a history of acute severe asthma or life-threatening anaphylactoid reactions should avoid precipitating agents. However, there are virtually no adequate controlled studies of the effect of salicylate and food additive avoidance in chronic asthma. *Tarlo and Broder* [160] did assess tartrazine and benzoate avoidance in 28 chronic asthmatics, 2 of whom reacted to tartrazine or benzoate provocation and 2 to ASA provocation (although a further 8 had a history of analgesic sensitivity but were not challenged). Only 1 patient improved over 1 month on the diet, and several actually worsened. However, the degree of sensitivity of most of their patients is uncertain and 1 required 300 mg ASA to produce a response on provocation. Those of our patients, whose severe unstable asthma has come under control on aspirin-additive avoidance, have been exquisitely sensitive and have experienced marked reactions after 1–50 mg of ASA. Another predictable variable in the response to dietary management is the individual patient's previous daily intake of the relevant substances.

ASA desensitization provides a potential alternative therapy. Repeated administration of a dose of ASA which initially produced symptoms leads to a refractory state [175]. This unresponsiveness can last for 5–7 days [118]. ASA-refractory patients do tolerate other NSAIDs [118], but it is not clear whether they also tolerate substances such as tartrazine. Maintenance of a refractory state by daily ASA administration has been used therapeutically [7, 27, 154]. However, even though most ASA-intolerant asthmatics improve with such measures, a significant number deteriorate [27]. Hopefully, elucidation of the pathophysiological mechanisms of this interesting syndrome will facilitate a more rational approach to its therapy.

Sensitivity to Sulphur Dioxide and Metabisulphites

Inhalation of sulphur dioxide has been shown to produce bronchoconstriction in experimental animals [109] and healthy men [59]. Exacerbations of pulmonary disorders by atmospheres contaminated by sulphur dioxide have been recognized for almost 2,000 years [60] and several epidemiological studies have shown that the symptomatic severity of asthma can be correlated with atmospheric sulphur dioxide pollution [95, 174]. Inhalation of sulphur dioxide has been shown to produce significant bronchoconstriction at 1 ppm in groups of asthmatics [83, 146]. Atopic adolescents without clinical asthma but with hyperreactive airways have a 3 to 22 times greater bronchospastic response to inhaled SO_2 than normal adolescents [85]. SO_2 also potentiates other bronchospastic responses [84]. The available evidence suggests that these effects are the result of an exaggerated vagal response to a chemical irritant on the background of general asthmatic bronchial hyperreactivity [20].

Despite the above, problems with sulphur dioxide in foods were not appreciated until 1977, when *Freedman* [60] demonstrated that asthmatics would also react to the sulphur dioxide contained in drinks. He found that 11% of asthmatics gave a history of reacting to soft drinks on routine questioning. 8 of 10 such patients reacted to provocation with 25 ml of an aqueous mixture of sodium metabisulphite and citric acid which yielded 100 ppm of sulphur dioxide, a concentration similar to that found in some brands of orange drinks. The air above such a mixture will have a greater than 1 ppm concentration of sulphur dioxide. The occurrence of bronchospasm within 1–2 min in *Freedman's* [60] patients suggests that the response was due to inhalation of the gas, or rapid absorption across the buccal mucosa.

Sodium and potassium bisulphite and metabisulphites, which are converted into sulphur dioxide in solution, and sulphur dioxide itself, are employed for a variety of purposes in food preparation, processing and storage. They are used both to sanitize equipment and as selective inhibitors of undesirable microorganisms in fermentation. They are used as antibacterial preservatives and as inhibitors of enzymic and non-enzymic discolouration in foods and are sometimes sprayed onto fresh fruit, vegetables and shellfish. Quite large amounts may be ingested with certain beers and wines (particularly home-fermented) and pre-prepared 'fresh' food meals in restaurants (such as vegetable and fruit salads).

4 cases reported by *Stevenson and Simon* [155] suggest that these sulphiting agents may produce anaphylactoid reactions by means other than the inhalation of released sulphur dioxide. Each of these patients had had severe reactions, with cyanosis, shock and even coma, after eating restaurant meals (such as salads) which would have contained sulphites. There was no evidence that these patients were allergic to the natural food. In each case, oral provocation with encapsulated potassium metabisulphite produced systemic and hypotensive symptoms as well as asthma. The mechanism of this reaction remains uncertain; these patients had negative potassium metabisulphite skin tests, but each did give histories of asthma provoked by irritant fumes and smog. Other reports confirm that wheezy dyspnoea, angioedema and abdominal symptoms can be produced by metabisulphites [120, 141] and it seems probable that further investigation will show this to be a common problem.

Non-Specific Histamine Release and Exogenous Histamine

Several of the foods most commonly incriminated in adverse reactions in atopic humans have been described as having non-specific histamine-releasing properties in some species of animal. These include egg-white, extracts of shellfish (both molluscs and crustacea), strawberries and some nuts [116, 139, 140]. Skin testing cannot differentiate between antibody-dependent and antibody-independent causes of mast cell mediator release, but the radio-allergosorbent test (RAST) does indicate true IgE-mediated allergy in many patients reacting to these foods [1, 28, 91]. Absence of circulating reagins in other cases does not prove the non-immunological nature of the reaction, since locally-produced IgE fixed to mast cells can produce local sensitization without entering the circulation [24, 73]. There is little direct evidence to incriminate non-specific histamine release as a common cause of clinical reactions to ingested rather than injected food in man.

Some foods and drinks, particularly when fermented or canned, contain significant amounts of histamine and other amines [121]. For example, more than 1 mg of histamine can be found per gram of certain cheeses. However, in healthy subjects a number of mechanisms, including mucosal diamine oxidases, inhibit significant absorption of histamine [86, 97]. The small amounts able to enter the portal vein are prevented from reaching the systemic circulation by hepatic metabolism [93]. Up to 2.75 mg/kg introduced duodenally is innocuous in healthy subjects and 165–200 mg will produce only brief facial flushing [106]. Certainly, foods containing histamine and putative histamine releasers are eaten without ill-effect by the vast majority of the population.

Moneret-Vautrin [106, 107] has suggested that histamine releasers, exogenous histamine in food, or histamine produced by the action of intestinal flora on high starch loads, can produce symptoms if the function of the intestinal mucosa is impaired by disease, or by the action of other substances which increase gut permeability. She has stated that, under such circumstances, duodenal instillation of histamine produces headache, urticaria and diarrhoea with significant elevations of peripheral histamine. This is surprising in view of the rapid systemic degradation of histamine, and has yet to be substantiated by independent experimental evidence.

Many patients with eczema have increased mucosal permeability [75] and changes in gut permeability can be demonstrated during local immune reactions in experimental animals [16, 21]. It does seem possible that systemic symptoms could be produced by large quantities of histamine releasers, or other vasoactive substances, in subjects with mucosal permeability changes due to gastrointestinal disease, or to co-existent local allergy to foods taken at the same meal. This mechanism remains hypothetical at the present time, but it would seem reasonable that a history suggesting it should instigate a review of any drugs taken by the patient which might increase mucosal permeability, and consideration of potential underlying gastrointestinal disease.

Pseudo-Allergy

Neurological and Psychological Changes Associated with Atopy

The most contentious issues in food hypersensitivity concern its supposed role in non-atopic somatic syndromes and in the genesis of psychological symptoms. Interactions between atopic symptoms and the psychological state are complex. Although the role of inhalant and food allergies in conditions such as asthma and eczema are well recognized, few would not also accept that they may be influenced by psychological factors. Information concerning non-specific bronchial hyperreactivity [68] and autonomic dysfunctions [158, 159] in atopy provide biochemical explanations of how any form of stress can induce a bronchospastic response in predisposed individuals. There is even objective evidence that exercise-induced asthma can be modified by hypnosis [12].

Any severe physical disorder can produce psychological distress, or lead to problems which could be classified as psychiatric disturbance. There are multiple reports describing emotional and neurotic difficulties in atopic children and adults [2, 15, 50, 61, 62, 72, 89, 149, 163, 169, 173]. However, there is no evidence that these symptoms predipose to atopic disorders and since they are symptoms which also occur in other physical disorders it is most likely that they are understandable reactions to the disorders or to their social consequences [54, 66, 103, 112, 114]. Children and adults with disfiguring eczema are often shunned by their peers. Many asthmatics are unable to take part in exertional pursuits. Episodes of life-threatening anaphylaxis or breathlessness induce anxiety or even fear in the most well-balanced patient or parent. One need not be surprised if a child behaves abnormally after spending all night scratching his eczema, or at 'temper tantrums' in an infant with undiagnosed milk-induced colic.

Allergic diseases can certainly produce neurological dysfunctions, which may be associated with mental changes. There are multiple reports of focal neurological signs, with or without psychological symptoms, in the course of angioedema and anaphylaxis [35, 78, 80, 115, 150, 165]. However, identical changes can be observed after any form of shock producing hypoxic cerebral injury. Focal neurological signs are also seen when cranial blood vessels are involved in any generalized vasculitis and have been reported after reactions to heterologous antisera [8, 79]. Similarly even relatively mild hypoxia can cause emotional lability and reduced intellectual function. In more severe degrees it may lead to overt confusional states and coma. It is not necessary to postulate a direct effect of allergy on the brain to explain such changes in asthma. However, a single case quoted from the Swedish literature of 1937 [22] does suggest the possibility of a more direct genesis of cerebral dysfunction in allergy: raised cerebrospinal fluid (CSF) pressure with CSF eosinophilia was found during a patient's reaction to fish, which took the form of somnolence, aphonia and nuchal rigidity, associated with skin erythema.

In the above situations psychological changes can be explained either as understandable secondary responses to physical or social difficulties, or as features of an acute organic reaction. However, more recently, claims have been made that psychiatric disturbances in general and multiple non-atopic somatic complaints are commonly (or even usually) the direct result of food allergy, even when not associated with features of the atopic syndrome.

There are several problems in attempting to evaluate these more recent claims. Firstly, they tend to have been put before the public in popular books [96, 128], magazines and radio and television programmes, rather than presented in scientific journals. Secondly, publications aimed at a more professional audience [39, 149], which do contain such statements, usually summarize the authors' clinical experience and opinions rather than provide the data on which they are based. In addition, the most crucial references are often found to be other summarized opinions, papers submitted for publication, abstracts of verbal communications, or publications of questionable relevance to that particular question. Many of the proclamations on this subject contain observations concerning atopic disease which would be accepted as valid by orthodox allergists, but which are extrapolated to inapplicable situations. Sometimes one can seriously question the validity of the logic by which these conclusions are drawn. A third major problem is the heterogeneity of the theories and practices of those diagnosing and treating 'allergy'. It is evident that even within the group describing themselves as clinical ecologists are practitioners who have adopted very individual blends of philosophies and diagnostic techniques (which range from orthodox skin testing to various more controversial clinical provocation and laboratory tests). The form of the subsequent therapy, the efficacy of which is said to justify the diagnosis, is often equally individual.

Many of the present claims concerning the importance and frequency of food allergy in psychiatric and non-atopic somatic conditions are very similar to, or are developments of, ideas initially put forward by workers such as *Rowe* and *Rinkel* in the 1920s and 1930s. Although many valid observations of true food allergy were indubitably made during that period, it is now equally clear that we must reassess conclusions reached at a time when there was considerable confusion regarding immunological mechanisms, the value of diagnostic tests, the power of the placebo effect, and before the need for blind provocation procedures was appreciated. Therefore we need to consider the evidence concerning the place of diagnostic techniques in the diagnosis of food allergy, and the history of the development of the major unorthodox positions, before considering the present situation.

Diagnosis of Food Hypersensitivity and Ancillary Tests

Double-Blind Food Provocation

Experiments utilizing double-blind food provocation techniques were first described in 1950. *Graham* et al. [67] showed that four doctors, who were convinced their migraine was due to chocolate, had no more headaches with chocolate than with placebo given blind. They also showed that urticarial lesions and measurable changes in skin blood flow could be induced by discussion of stressful events or of circumstances associated with previous attacks of urticaria. Nasal hypersecretion and eosinophilia, chest and abdominal symptoms, and measurable changes in gastrointestinal motility, could all be induced by telling patients they had been given a food to which they believed themselves allergic, even though the same patients did not respond to the food when they were unaware that they had had it.

A vast experience with suggestion, hypnosis and controlled drug trials since 1950 has confirmed that virtually any physical or mental symptom can be induced by the 'placebo effect'. Few people will not have experienced revulsion, nausea and possibly other symptoms on contemplating eating a substance to which they have a particular aversion, whether or not they have ever actually eaten it. In a recent review, *Lessof* [90] has asserted that the most common cause of an aversion to food is in fact psychological. Our own experiments certainly indicate that psychological reactions are common in some patient groups [11, 117]. Double-blind provocation only confirms the presence of organic hypersensitivity in about a third of asthmatic children giving histories of food-induced symptoms [100]. At present, some form of double-blind feeding test is the only means of proving clinically relevant organic intolerance and until some other test has been shown as effective it must remain the yardstick by which other techniques are judged [17, 101]. The frequency of psychological reactions also means that any conclusions drawn about food hypersensitivity or allergy diagnosed without double-blind confirmation must be viewed with considerable circumspection.

Regrettably it is only recently that double-blind provocation techniques have been used at all commonly to avoid the influences of suggestion and observer bias on the investigation of food allergy. Foods have been administered double-blind using nasogastric tubes [58], food disguised in soups [23], gruels or pseudo-'milk shakes' [117], and by placing freeze-dried foods in opaque capsules [13, 100, 117]. Administration by nasogastric tube and encapsulation have been criticized because they by-pass the buccal mucosa as a potential site of antigen absorption. However, the administration of food in capsules has been shown to elicit reproducible reactions in atopic children [17, 100] and adults [13].

RAST and Skin Testing

In the presence of double-blind confirmed hypersensitivity, positive skin prick tests, or demonstration of circulating antibodies of IgE class, provide circumstantial evidence that the reaction is immunological. These and other techniques have also been used to diagnose food allergy. Skin reactions to locally-introduced allergens had been described by *Blackley* [14] in 1873 and many of the essential features of scratch testing relevant to food hypersensitivity were described by *Schloss* [142, 143] between 1912 and 1920, who established that adverse reactions to foods could occur with negative skin tests and that positive skin tests could be found in the absence of clinical hypersensitivity.

Intradermal skin testing came to be used widely after its adoption by some influential American allergists in the 1920s. This was probably related in part to misunderstanding of what *Schloss* described as 'false-positive' and 'false-negative' results and in part to a wish to find a technique which would provide some confirmation of clinical impressions concerning the frequency of food hypersensitivity. Intradermal skin tests are frequently positive when scratch, or prick/puncture tests are negative as they may detect lower levels of tissue sensitization [19]. Hence they may have a lower incidence of apparent 'false-negatives'. It is difficult to be certain to what extent individual allergists accepted the results of skin testing alone as diagnostic over the next 30 years. However, it is evident that many did consider any positive result as highly suggestive of clinical hypersensitivity, and as adequate confirmation of their subjective impressions.

Modern appreciation of the non-immunological nature of some adverse reactions and of the biology of IgE provide a clearer theoretical base for the assessment of skin tests and techniques for measurement of circulating antibodies. From information concerning local mucosal IgE-antibody production and mast cell fixation, and of other local defence mechanisms, one would predict the occurrence both of local hypersensitivity without positive skin tests or RAST, and of positive tests without clinical hypersensitivity. Also one can now appreciate that allergic reactions are not all-or-nothing responses: reactions great enough to be observed clinically will depend both on the level of tissue sensitization with antibody and the dosage of food ingested.

Recently, double-blind provocation tests have been used to reassess skin prick and intradermal tests in a large series of asthmatic children with histories of adverse reactions to foods [18, 19, 100]; it was found that all children with confirmable clinical sensitivity to foods had positive skin tests. However, only about half the children who had positive prick tests to the foods which most commonly produced clinical reactions, actually reacted to those foods on double blind provocation. Several foods were found never to produce clinical reactions. although positive skin prick tests to them were common. Intradermal skin tests were found to be considerably less efficient in predicting the response to double blind provocation. No patients were identified who reacted clinically, but who had a positive intradermal skin test and a negative prick test; and individual foods produced positive intradermal tests in the absence of clinical reactions in between 18 and 46% of the patients. It should be noted that patients from this series, who had negative double blind provocation tests, could then tolerate the same food given openly. This suggests that double blind provocation itself does not give 'false-negatives', as well as demonstrating the unreliability of clear histories of reactions even in highly atopic individuals.

Despite the above, other recent workers have confirmed that hypersensitivity reactions to foods can occur, at least in atopic adults, in the absence of positive skin prick tests. It is uncertain whether this is because of sensitization limited to a single organ; because the reactions are not IgE mediated; or because some commercially available reagents are inadequate. *Lessof* et al. [91] found positive prick tests or RAST to milk in only 30% of patients they considered to have organic milk intolerance on the basis of several criteria which did not always include double blind provocation. *Bernstein* et al. [13] found only a 30% correlation between the results of skin prick tests and double blind food provocation in 22 adults with a history suggestive of IgE-mediated food sensitivity. We have not only seen negative prick tests to milk in atopic adults with double blind-proven hypersensitivity, but have also seen food skin tests become positive only after starting exclusion of the relevant food [11].

Measurement of specific circulating antibodies of IgE class by RAST has a reasonable correlation with the results of skin prick and provocation tests to inhalant antigens [1, 10, 24, 28, 171]. However, RAST correlates less well with clinical history of food sensitivity than prick tests [28]. Like skin prick testing, RAST is more reliable with regard to fish, pear, nuts and egg and can be misleading in the case of cereals and milk [1]. We are unaware of any published study in which the role of RAST in the diagnosis of food allergy has been assessed specifically and systematically using double blind provocation testing. However, the study of *Bernstein* et al. [13] demonstrated positive RAST with negative provocation tests and positive double blind food provocations with negative RASTs. Some reports suggest that the combined use of skin prick testing and RAST has advantages over the use of either technique used alone [1, 28, 91].

Subcutaneous and Sublingual Provocation Testing

The rationale behind RAST testing, skin prick and intradermal testing is the detection of circulating, or tissue-fixed specific antibody of IgE class. Several other techniques have been described which have a less secure scientific foundation. Subcutaneous provocation-neutralization testing was described by *Lee* [87] in 1961. In this test a sufficient quantity of food extract to elicit the patient's presenting complaints is injected subcutaneously. The injection of a higher dilution of the same extract should then relieve the symptoms. The similar sublingual test was initially described in 1944. In one of the commoner variations of this method [108], several drops of extract are placed under the tongue of the patient. When symptoms appear they should be 'turned off' by a more dilute sublingual dose. It is claimed that symptoms due to ingestion of the relevant food will be prevented if the 'neutralizing dose' established by this means is administered sublingually before meals.

Anaphylaxis after antigen injection, and the immediate oral itching and swelling after chewing food in genuinely hypersensitive patients, demonstrate that these routes of administration can indeed provoke symptoms. However, the only evidence to support the use of either of these forms of provocation testing in routine diagnosis is anecdotal, or open to criticism of the study design. Both have been subjected to numerous double blind evaluations [reviewed in 29, 53] which have failed to find evidence to support their efficacy in either diagnosis or treatment. In one such investigation by *Kailin and Collier* [77], 5 physicians who had been using the method for at least 7 years were allowed to choose patients known to react, but no distinction could be made between active and placebo preparations on repeat double blind testing. In a more recent double blind study, *Lehman* [88] also reported that changes in symptoms and signs occurred as frequently after placebo as after sublingual food extract administration.

Various forms of cytotoxicity testing in which circulating white blood cells are exposed in vitro to food extracts have been advocated since 1947. Several objective studies have also failed to find evidence that this form of testing is effective in the diagnosis of food or inhalant allergy [53].

In position statements on controversial techniques made by the American Academy of Allergy [53] in 1981, it was advised that, as the available evidence indicated that sublingual and subcutaneous provocation methods were ineffective, and cytotoxicity testing was unproven, these techniques should be reserved for experimental use, and then only in properly designed trials.

In summary, all the available evidence demonstrates that double blind feeding is the only test which reliably indicates the presence or absence of clinically relevant sensitivity to food, although skin prick testing and RAST may have a useful ancillary role. Consequently, studies in which diagnoses of food hypersensitivity have been based on other techniques, such as sublingual or subcutaneous provocation testing, must be viewed with considerable circumspection.

Historical Development of Theories Concerning Food Allergy in Non-Atopic Conditions

Many of the very early papers on food allergy are models of clinical observation and concerned anaphylactic reactions, which today would be considered typical of IgE-mediated atopic disease. The association of such reactions with the other features of the atopic syndrome was recognized by 1916 [30]. From then to the 1930s many articles appeared incriminating food allergy as a cause of a wide variety of complaints in addition to the better recognized features of the atopic syndrome. Most reports were of individual cases or small groups of patients, most of whom did have other associated allergic symptoms. Upper and lower gastrointestinal symptoms, including cyclical vomiting; neurological dysfunctions including migraine and epilepsy; muscle and joint symptoms, including arthritis; scattered spasms and pains; and possibly psychological symptoms such as vague feelings of ill health and fatigue, apathy, dullness, excitement and hyperactivity were all attributed to food allergy on an anecdotal basis [3, 4, 48, 49, 52, 72, 137, 166].

Rowe [136, 137], recognizing the limitations of skin testing, devised elimination diets which are still influential. His diagnoses of food allergy were based on relief of symptoms on exclusion diets, sometimes supported by skin tests. Occasionally he described return of the symptoms when patients deviated from their diets. Although the majority of the 175 food allergic patients described by him in 1928 [136] had major atopic manifestations, by 1930 he had become convinced that 'allergy' was responsible for many vague subjective, chronic symptoms. Almost a third of the patients described by him in 1931 [137] had symptoms which could be related to psychological disturbance and approximately 20 had overtly psychological symptoms including nervousness, depression, lack of confidence, irritability, mental lassitude, difficulty in remembering, concentrating and thinking, etc. However, from *Rowe's* own descriptions, the mental changes in many of his patients would now be considered to be probably secondary to the processes discussed earlier, rather than to a direct effect of allergy on the brain.

Rinkel's concepts of 'masked' and 'cyclical' allergies were developed in the 1930s. Although using skin tests, *Rinkel* [130] described his diagnoses of food allergy as being based mainly on his clinical experience, supported by food exclusion and open reintroduction. According to this theory, allergies may be 'fixed' (usually associated with positive skin tests) or 'cyclical' (often with negative skin tests). The sensitivity in cyclical allergy is reputedly dependent on how often a particular food is eaten: the more frequently it is eaten the greater the sensitivity. However, a food eaten every day may not be recognized as deleterious at this stage of the cycle because it initially relieves the symptoms which were the result of the previous ingestion. This is the stage of 'masked allergy'. If that food is excluded for increasing periods of time, the patient will go through several further stages: First, the patient will become more sensitive (active allergy), so that a single exposure will produce severe symptoms. Later, the patient will become less sensitive (latent allergy) so that symptoms will only follow the second or third feeding in several days. Finally, with more prolonged exposure he will become tolerant. However, according to this concept, reintroduction of the food on a daily basis will produce a return through the steps of latent, active and masked allergy and all 'allergics' will tend to become sensitive to any foods eaten every day.

Although some of *Rinkel's* later applications of skin test titration methods [131] and subcutaneous provocation testing [132] have since been highly criticized, it must be remembered that he, like *Rowe,* was working predominantly with atopic patients. His theories were almost certainly an attempt to explain some of the then more confusing aspects of genuine hypersensitivity (many of which are now explicable in the light of knowledge concerning IgE and mast cell physiology) such as the period of anergy which may follow anaphylactic episodes; and the effects of different frequencies of antigen exposure in increasing or decreasing degrees of IgE-mediated sensitivity.

Rinkel's concepts of masked and cyclical allergy were later expanded by others and applied in a much wider setting. *Randolph* [123, 127] introduced the idea that the masking phenomenon leads directly to behavioural changes by producing a craving for the food to which the individual is sensitive: 'addiction' to the food results because the food relieves the symptoms produced by the previous ingestion, or even produces a supranormal sense of well-being. *Randolph* [125, 127] then linked these concepts to *Selye's* [145] work on the physiology of adaptation to produce a much more general philosophy of maladaptation to the total environment.

Randolph [127] likens an initial stage of reacting to 'toxic' agents to the physiological alarm reaction. Repeated exposure supposedly leads to an adaptation stage with apparent tolerance, but in which the individual is actually addicted to the harmful agent. As this stage progresses the individual requires larger and more frequent doses of the food to avoid withdrawal symptoms. Finally the ability of the organism to maintain adaptation is overwhelmed so that the stage recurs in which acute post-exposure symptoms are seen. This is likened to the exhaustion stage of the general adaptation syndrome. According to *Randolph,* with increasing sensitivity, and with increasing dosages, eating the food in the addiction stage leads to increasing mental stimulation, progressing up to mania with or without convulsions. The withdrawal effects progress through local allergic manifestations, then systemic allergic manifestations, disturbed mentation and finally severe depression with or without disturbed consciousness.

Although *Randolph* has claimed that this theory has 'opened up an ecologic approach to mental illness', the type of mental disturbance he describes bears only slight resemblance to manic-depressive illness as it is recognized by psychiatrists. In particular, muscle twitching, jerking of the extremities, convulsive seizures and altered consciousness are not features of mania. Nor are typical atopic features usually encountered at the onset of the depressive phase. If such features were to be encountered, the phenomenological diagnosis would be an acute organic reaction, not an affective psychosis, and appropriate investigations instituted to make an aetiological diagnosis. It is perhaps surprising that in the 30 years since *Randolph* put forward his theory and despite having tested 'thousands of patients . . . tens of thousands of times during the past three decades', he has failed to document in an accepted neurological or psychiatric journal, any series of manic-depressive patients, or series of patients with atypical affective psychoses or acute organic reactions, in which food has been demonstrated to be an aetiological factor.

Randolph's maladaptation theory has been taken a step further by some clinical ecologists who maintain that psychological symptoms in response to social stress are not 'neurotic' (i.e. the result of psychodynamic factors, or learned behavioural patterns), but are the direct result of food allergies induced by a breakdown in adaptation to the total physical and social environment [5]. On this basis they appear to consider that treatment of the allergies is more important than any type of psychotherapy, or intervention in the psychosocial factors which led to the symptoms.

The nature of these theories as they are now put forward, and their predictions, are such that it is very difficult to see how any objective data could be obtained which could either prove, or disprove them. They appear to be held as a quasi-scientific, philosophical belief system by some, who choose to interpret disparate and otherwise unrelated scientific findings in their support. At the same time any work which fails to confirm the theory is dismissed as, ipso facto, of faulty design or execution: and those who do not accept it are accused of narrow-mindedly refusing to accept the self-evident. *Randolph* [124] himself stresses that the principles of holistic medicine and clinical ecology are reached by a process of reasoning (described as 'inductive') which differs from that employed in conventional academic medicine.

Clinical Evidence Concerning Psychological and Emotional Changes Due To Allergy

We have already noted that neurological complications of anaphylaxis, mental changes due to hypoxia in asthmatics, and behavioural and emotional abnormalities in both children and adults with prolonged atopic physical problems are well documented. Although such observations have been taken to support a direct role for allergy in the generation of mental symptoms, we have also noted that they could be adequately explained by other physical and psychodynamic factors. Although clinical ecologists such as *Randolph* incriminate food in virtually all abnormal behaviours that others might describe as neurotic or psychotic, three more or less specific psychiatric syndromes have been attributed to food hypersensitivity or allergy: the 'allergic tension-fatigue syndrome', hyperactivity (both predominantly in children), and schizophrenia.

Allergic Tension-Fatigue Syndrome

Speer [149] has defined a set of personality characteristics and behavioural traits, which he believes characteristic of patients with multiple allergies, as the 'allergic tension-fatigue syndrome'. He states that these would usually be considered as an exaggeration of a normal pattern rather than one which would ordinarily be called abnormal or pathological. *Allergic tension* is a very general inclination to overdo and overreact, which *Speer* sees as responsible for several different behaviour patterns, from high drive and dynamism leading to success in the world; to anxiety, vague forebodings of unknown future calamity and marked timidity. He considers *allergic fatigue* as a counterreaction to this tension and uses the term to describe various subjective feelings of general malaise, most of which could be interpreted by others as features of anxiety or depression.

Speer [149] described this syndrome as occurring in patients with allergic diseases such as asthma, eczema and rhinitis. While accepting that it may in part represent a secondary reaction to the distress of these conditions, he states categorically that 'all highly allergic patients display some evidence of this distressing condition' and 'the allergic tension-fatigue syndrome may occur as a primary allergic disease, not necessarily accompanied by other signs of allergy'. He quotes no evidence other than experience to support these statements, yet his monograph [149] is often quoted in clinical ecology publications as authority for the view that allergy is a direct cause of neurotic symptoms. A major part of this book concerns encephalomyelitic reactions to vaccines, the Guillain-Barré syndrome and the neurological complications of conditions associated with vasculitis such as serum sickness and lupus erythematosus. These are used as general circumstantial evidence incriminating 'allergy' in mental and neurological problems.

There are 2 cases in the literature in which the allergic-tension fatigue syndrome has been reported to have been induced by double blind feeding. In both cases mental symptoms could have been secondary to physical problems. *Crook* et al. [34] described a child who was tired and irritable with headaches and abdominal pain. These symptoms recurred 3 days after commencing blind milk reintroduction and ceased 48 h after stopping tablets containing milk. *Rapp* [129] reported a 9-year-old child who was very tired and irritable and who had allergic rhinitis and conjunctivitis. Milk provocation produced puffy eyes and nasal congestion as well as irritability within 2 h.

Hyperactivity in Children

Feingold [55] and *Feingold* et al. [57] have proposed that hyperactive behaviour in children (hyperkinesis) is associated with the ingestion of salicylates and the other common cross-reacting food additives. They noted that an adult patient with ASA intolerance had shown remission of psychiatric disturbances when on a diet free of salicylates, preservatives and colouring agents; and had correlated increased consumption of food additives with a reported increasing incidence of hyperkinetic-learning disabled children. He subsequently reported that 30–50% of hyperactive children in his practice had a complete remission of symptoms on a salicylate and additive-free diet [56].

Feingold's claims received considerable publicity and public support, particularly in the USA, following several oral presentations, a popular book and testimony in the US Congressional record. Multiple criticisms of his work were raised immediately [9], which in summary stated that his claims were impressionistic, anecdotal and lacking in objective evidence [110]. Several controlled studies have since been performed to test this hypothesis. Most have failed to support a significant effect of diet on hyperactive behaviour [51, 69, 98, 111, 161]. However, the results of two authoritative studies provide limited support for the Feingold theory: *Weiss* et al. [168] found a deterioration of behaviour in only 2 of 22 hyperactive children challenged with a mixture of food dyes after 3 months on an additive-free diet. *Swanson and Kinsbourne* [157] found that the administration of food dyes impaired the performance of hyperactive children on a laboratory learning test. However, these studies have been criticized both in terms of design and the interpretation of results [170]. In relation to the latter study [157] it is important to note that no *behavioural* response to the dyes was documented by the rating scale employed. A comparison of diet and stimulant medications has shown that overall, drugs are considerably more effective than diet in controlling hyperactive behaviour [172].

Public interest in, and controversy concerning, the Feingold hypothesis has been so great that the US National Institutes of Health convened a 'consensus development conference' to evaluate the evidence [111]. This concluded that the bulk of the evidence does not support the

Feingold hypothesis, although it does not exclude the possibility that hyperactive behaviour could be attributable to food dyes in a minority of cases. It is perhaps unfortunate that many of the controlled studies designed specifically to test the Feingold hypothesis have tended to ignore other coincident hypersensitivity responses and the possibility that effects on behaviour could be secondary to these. *Warner* [167] has reported a child, in whom double blind colour provocation induced acute urticaria and behavioural changes: although the mother considered the child hyperactive, she had not recognized that it had been suffering from chronic urticaria.

Schizophrenia

Dohan's work has been interpreted as implying the involvement of food allergy in the production of schizophrenia. *Dohan* [44] actually suggested that the basic biological defect in schizophrenia is a genetic impairment of the gut and other barrier systems which permits the passage of cereal-derived neuroactive peptides from the gut lumen to the brain cells. In support of this gluten hypothesis he has drawn upon histological, biochemical and clinical observations of others, marshalled with epidemiological, immunopathological and clinical evidence of his own. The link between some of these strands of evidence is their supposed support for a relationship between coeliac disease and schizophrenia.

Dohan's [43] claim that there is a relationship between schizophrenia and coeliac disease is based upon his belief that schizophrenics have small intestinal abnormalities characteristic of coeliac disease, that the two conditions occur in the same person more commonly than would be expected by chance, and that the ingestion of gluten by coeliac patients can result in psychosis. However, two large studies have failed to find evidence of coeliac disease in schizophrenics [36, 152], three out of four of the studies regarded by *Dohan* as demonstrating a more than coincidental association of coeliac disease and schizophrenia concern childhood psychosis rather than schizophrenia, and none of the studies quoted by him contains a convincing account of schizophrenia occurring in a patient with coeliac disease.

The epidemiological evidence which *Dohan* cites are the apparent correlations between the fall in hospital admission rates for schizophrenia during World War II and the severity of rationing [41] and fall in wheat consumption, plus a correlation of 'morbid risk' for schizophrenia in various countries and the extent to which wheat features in the typical local diet [42]. The first two correlations could reflect some other effect of wartime conditions. The reported correlation of 'morbid risk' for schizophrenia and diet between countries is puzzling in the light of other evidence that rates for schizophrenia are fairly constant from one country to another [32]. It is possible that the differences in 'morbid risk' which *Dohan* quotes are simply a reflection of different measuring instruments and diagnostic criteria in the countries to which he refers.

A number of dietary studies have been carried out to test the hypothesis. Although three [46, 47, 147] have appeared to support the usefulness of gluten-free diets in schizophrenics the 'blindness' of the gluten challenges has to be questioned in view of the fact that patients receiving gluten supplements felt 'more full and satisfied' [156] and in one study the interviewer-rater may not have been blind [92]. The third study [147] has also been challenged on the grounds that the statistical analyses were inappropriate and that the subjects were atypical [92, 148]. Four other dietary trials have provided no support for the gluten hypothesis of schizophrenia [76, 113, 119, 156].

Immunopathological evidence quoted as supporting the gluten hypothesis are findings that 17–20% of schizophrenics have antibodies to wheat gliadin detected by enzyme-linked and latex conglutination techniques [70, 45], that antibodies to whole wheat and rye detected by indirect immunofluorescence are more common in schizophrenics than controls [71], and that 50% of schizophrenics have lymphocyte reactivity to gluten similar to that found in coeliac disease [6]. However, other studies using tanned red cells, microprecipitation, indirect immunofluorescence and RAST have failed to find differences in antibodies to wheat and gluten between schizophrenics and controls [82, 104, 133]. Lack of agreement between these studies could be due to the techniques employed, lack of blindness of laboratory staff in some studies, differences in selection criteria for schizophrenic and non-schizophrenic psychotic subjects, and the use of inappropriate control groups. Two studies which did employ similar diagnostic criteria for schizophrenic and affective psychoses, matched control groups from the same hospitals as the psychotics, and in one instance blind application of the laboratory tests [104, 133], failed to find evidence for a relationship between schizophrenia as a diagnosis, or schizophrenic symptoms, and antibodies to wheat or gluten.

For the time being, *Dohan's* hypothesis of a toxic effect of cereal-derived peptides in the genesis of schizophrenia must remain a hypothesis. The evidence in favour of it is not convincing and the fairest judgement is the Scottish legal verdict of 'not proven'. The only data which can be taken as supporting the hypothesis are circumstantial and do not provide any direct evidence to incriminate a role for allergic mechanisms in the generation of mental symptoms or psychosis.

Non-Specific Neurotic and Psychiatric Syndromes

In addition to the particular conditions discussed above, it has also been suggested that food allergy is a common direct cause of a whole range of psychiatric and associated somatic symptoms in various non-specific syndromes whether or not these are associated with other atopic conditions. *Speer* [149] stated that 'no patient should be classified as having a neurosis until allergy has been considered'. Claims of this nature have been popularized by books [96, 128]. In the latter, which 'is dedicated to all patients who have been called neurotic, hypochondriac, hysterical, or starved for attention, while actually suffering from environmentally induced illness', *Randolph and Moss* [128] assert that 'Allergies can not only cause familiar physical symptoms but can also be responsible for a host of so-called mental problems, including some cases of what look like outright psychoses'. Table II lists symptoms which are attributed to allergy by *Mac Karness* [96] and other clinical ecologists.

Very few of the almost 100 reports linking psychological changes to food hypersensitivity, which have appeared in the literature since 1922, have included any form of blind feeding experiments. The diagnosis of food hypersensitivity in most early reports depended on relief of symptoms on food exclusion, with or without exacerbation on open reintroduction. Many of the later authors on this subject, who have relied on diagnostic techniques of unproven efficacy such as sublingual provocation testing and pulse rate changes after open food reintroduction, discount the relevance of the placebo effect to food-induced symptoms. In a major text on clinical ecology, *Randolph* [126] states that suggestion is not a major factor in open testing and that blind controls are not required routinely because blind nasogastric feeding has confirmed reactions (of what type is not stated) in an adequate number of cases. The argument that because some sensitivities identified by a particular means can be confirmed, then all 'sensitivities' identified in that manner would be confirmed if subjected to blind testing is not supported by the evidence.

The attitude of some of those using subcutaneous or sublingual provocation testing in the diagnosis of food-induced mental changes is indicated by the statement included in a letter by *Glaisher* [64]: 'There is no need

Table II. Symptoms and conditions attributed to allergy by clinical ecologists

(a) Specific medical conditions [derived from 96]	
Bronchitis	Migraine
Conjunctivitis	Bell's palsy
Asthma	Epilepsy
Eczema	Vertigo
Urticaria	Neuroses
Rhinitis	Mania, hypomania
Aphthous ulcers	Depression
Peptic ulcers	Schizophrenia
Crohn's disease	Hypo- and hyperthyroidism
Ulcerative colitis	Infertility
Angina	Vaginal discharge
Hypertension	Dys- or amenorrhea
Intermittent claudication	Menorrhagia
Obesity	Arthritis
(b) Symptoms considered indicative of allergy [derived from publicity leaflet distributed to Manchester health-food stores]	
Persistent fatigue	Feeling faint
Obesity	Feeling unwell all over
Fluctuating weight	Terrible thoughts on waking
Water retention	Shaking in the morning
Swelling	Slow getting started
Palpitations	Crabby on waking
Slow or rapid heartbeat	Insomnia
Chest pain (particularly left sided)	Difficulty waking up
High blood pressure	Mood swings
Cramp in limbs	Irritability
Chilblains	Panic attacks
Dyspepsia, abdominal distress	Inability to think clearly
Flatulence	Feeling depersonalized
Abdominal bloating	Lack of confidence
Constipation	Undue elation
Diarrhoea	Low mood
Variability in bowel function	Generally slowing down
Nausea	Generally speeding up
Stiff throat or tongue	Excitement or silliness
Tingling all over	Tiredness after eating
Ringing in the ears	Feeling drained and exhausted
Giddiness	Impotence
Frequent urination	Frigidity
Headaches	Eating binges
Faints and fits	

for a double-blind trial in these patients. The demonstration is so clear cut and repeatable that one has to accept that allergy to foods plays a very great part in the production of depression and mania.' The only placebo-controlled series of an adequate number of patients tested in this way, which has apparently supported this contention, has been published by *King* [81]. 'Cognitive-emotional' symptoms were observed significantly more commonly after all antigen than all placebo sublingual administrations in new patients at a Connecticut Center for Bio-Ecologic Disease. However, the design was such that the patients could not have remained truly blind as to the identity of placebo provocations: the placebo was triple distilled water (to avoid the risk of biological reactions), whereas the antigens were standard extracts which taste of phenol even when the characteristic flavour of the food is not obvious. It is stated in this paper itself, that patients were frequently correct in identifying when they had been given water. It also appears that during this study, symptoms following placebo administrations were sometimes attributed by the investigator to previous administrations of allergen.

Apart from the reports quoted in earlier sections of this chapter the only published cases known to us in which blind feeding has been claimed to have produced psychological symptoms are those of *Finn and Cohen* [58], *Brown* et al. [23], *Denman* [38], and *Randolph and Moss* [128]. *Finn and Cohen* [58] reported 6 cases of patients with severe physical symptoms and either social or psychological problems which resolved on dietary exclusion and in 3 of whom physical symptoms were produced by nasogastric provocation. 5 of these cases had physical or 'mental' symptoms which could be accounted for by the known toxic effects of high doses of the xanthine derivatives contained in the tea or coffee considered responsible (i.e. palpatations, headache, nausea, nervousness, etc.). It was recorded that 3 of the patients usually ingested unusually large doses of these beverages. One self-professed 'tea fiend' was agoraphobic when having tea-induced supraventricular tachycardias, but returned to a normal social life following tea and coffee avoidance.

Brown et al. [23] studied 12 patients in whom open testing had incriminated one or more of several foods, of which grain, milk, egg, coffee and tea were the most common. Blind food provocation was performed by incorporating the challenge food in a pureed vegetable soup. Atopic status was not recorded and few details of the patients were given except that they had multiple symptoms and were similar to the patients described by *Finn and Cohen* [58]. 8 complained of depression, 8 of headache or migraine and 7 of bowel disturbance. Unspecified symptoms followed incriminated food provocations significantly more frequently than placebo provocations, in the group as a whole. However, only 3 of the patients reacted to each antigen preparation without reporting reactions to any of the placebos and 6 patients responded to 50% or more of the control provocations.

Only two descriptions of apparently psychotic behaviour induced by blind feeding are known to us. *Denman* [38] reported a 14-year-old girl who had milk-related gastrointestinal symptoms in childhood and who developed mental disturbance with bouts of crying, 'hysteria' and hearing voices when she lapsed from her milk-free diet. Double blind milk provocation induced a recurrence of physical and mental symptoms; and the reaction could be blocked by sodium cromoglycate. *Randolph and Moss* [128] described a 30-year-old woman whose headaches, and alternating hyperactivity and depression, improved on an elimination diet. On eating beets she became 'psychotic, racing for the exits, screaming, yelling and trying by every means to get out of the place. She was even leaning out of an eighth floor window . . . desperately seeking to get more air and apparently unaware of the danger of falling out'. With beet or beet juice given blindly by nasogastric tube she was 'again ... to all appearances, psychotic'.

In summary: there is abundant evidence that psychological and social problems can be secondary to the well-recognized physical effects of genuine allergic, and toxic pharmacological, reactions. There is no published objective evidence to support claims that multiple non-atopic somatic symptoms or psychological disorders are commonly the direct result of food hypersensitivity.

Recent Investigations in Food Allergy and Pseudo-Allergy

Lack of scientific method in arriving at new insights does not invalidate them. The history of medicine demonstrates that all advances were once considered unorthodox. However, many opinions, both orthodox and unorthodox, have since been shown to be invalid. History also demonstrates the dangers of the widespread adoption of treatments before they have been subjected to objective scientific appraisal. We considered that the implications of some of the claims regarding the role of food allergy in common physical and mental disorders were potentially enormous. We therefore set out to search for positive evidence to support them. To do this we based our methods on advice from colleagues who claimed to find a high incidence of food allergy; but also applied objective testing for organic food sensitivity in the form of double blind provocation and used standardized psychiatric techniques for the objective measurement of psychological changes.

We will mention the results of two of our studies here. Details of the methodology are published elsewhere [117]. Briefly, we attempted to identify food hypersensitivities by exclusion-reintroduction protocols followed by repeated open, and then double blind, provocation. Patients were also examined by an independent psychiatrist who also followed changes in psychological symptoms in the course of provocation tests. The aims of the studies were to look for objective evidence of food hypersensitivity in different clinical presentations; to examine the nature of food-induced somatic and psychological symptoms; and to compare both the medical and psychiatric features of patients with and without confirmable hypersensitivity. In the first study [117] we examined 23 consecutive patients who presented to an allergy clinic with a belief that they suffered from food allergy (excluding only patients who had chronic urticaria alone). In the second study [11] we examined 27 patients attending a gastroenterology clinic with persistent symptoms of the irritable bowel syndrome (IBS).

We could only find objectively-confirmable hypersensitivity in 4 of the 23 patients who considered they had food allergy when we first saw them. Each of these 4 had classical atopic disease and 3 had been aware of their food sensitivity since childhood. The fourth was a late-onset aspirin-sensitive asthmatic. All 4 had asthma (or have since developed it), allergic rhinitis and a history of acute urticaria. 2 of the patients had immediate oral itching and swelling followed by abdominal pain after eating the food. 3 had positive immediate skin prick tests to the relevant food. In our study of IBS we found 3 patients whose bowel symptoms responded to food exclusion and who had positive double blind provocation tests. Each of these patients was also highly atopic: all having allergic rhinitis, 2 asthma and 2 atopic eczema. Psychological changes in the course of reactions to food provocation tests were not seen in any of the patients with confirmed hypersensitivity from either study.

We were unable to find positive evidence to support the presence of food hypersensitivity in 19 of the 23 patients who had presented believing they had food allergy. In 14 we believed the results of food exclusion and double blind provocation had reasonably excluded this diagnosis.

Table III. Symptoms attributed to food allergy in patients without objectively confirmable organic food hypersensitivity[1] [from ref. 117]

Lethargy, tiredness, being vaguely 'not well'
Sleep disturbance, daytime or post-prandial drowsiness
Head, abdominal, chest, joint and muscle pains
Nausea, abdominal swelling and/or discomfort; constipation and/or diarrhoea
Breathlessness, palpitations, dizziness, lightheadedness, faints
Parasthesiae, itching or burning skin, peripheral 'swelling'
Poor concentration, disorientation, loss of memory and/or confidence
Depression, irritability, mood swings, panic attacks, agoraphobia
Disturbed sexual function

[1] 19 patients, with an average of more than 6 presenting complaints each.

5 patients had to be classified as not fully assessable allergologically because of their refusal to comply with all the conditions of the study. However, since the available evidence indicated that hypersensitivity was unlikely in all but 1 of the latter, and since the only difference between the two subgroups was in the degree of their poor compliance, these 19 patients were subsequently considered as one group with 'unconfirmable food allergy'.

The symptoms of the patients with unconfirmable allergy are shown in table III. As can be seen they show a very similar symptom profile to many patients considered to have food allergy by *Rowe* [137], *MacKarness* [96] and others. All of these patients attributed overtly psychological symptoms, as well as somatic complaints, to their presumed allergy. Although several had symptoms which can occur in atopic disease and 6 could have been considered atopic on the basis of previous personal history, family history and skin tests, evidence of bronchoconstriction was not found in those complaining of episodic breathlessness, nor was urticaria seen in those complaining of itching. In addition, œdema was not found in those complaining of peripheral swelling.

These patients were considerably more difficult to investigate than those presenting with classical atopic conditions. Although polysymptomatic and sometimes bringing lists of their symptoms, they tended to be vague about the details of their histories, concentrating more on the effects their illness had on their lives. They co-operated poorly with the investigations, frequently finding excuses for not completing dietary and provocation studies, or performing them in a manner which made proper interpretation of the results impossible. Even those who appeared totally confident of their ability to identify a particular food tended to become vague or evasive about their subjective responses to double blind provocations. Some became hostile if pressed to decide whether or not they had experienced a reaction.

Most of these patients thought they had identified offending foods by various means, including self-administered exclusion diets, before they attended our clinic. However, several believed they must have unidentified allergies and were unaware of any specific food-symptom associations. When advised not to consider themselves sensitive unless they reacted to all of three open reintroductions, most came to tolerate at least some previously avoided foods. No patients from this group had positive double blind provocations with food. In 7 patients the occurrence of reactions on every occasion a food was given openly, which were not reproduced on double blind administration, suggested the presence of psychogenic reactions. In addition, all but 1 of these patients reported reactions to more than one of the placebos on each double blind series of 6 provocations, even though they tolerated the same substances used as placebos when these were given openly. Marked fluctuations in psychological symptoms were seen frequently in the course of food exclusions and open reintroductions, but no consistent psychological-symptom responses to blind food administrations could be found.

Our studies do not provide any evidence that psychological or other somatic symptoms not generally associated with classical atopy are caused directly by food hypersensitivity. Psychological symptoms were not observed in the course of organic reactions to foods, and food hypersensitivity could not be confirmed in any patient with a non-atopic presentation. However, in 1 patient from our IBS study, there was evidence to suggest that psychological symptoms were secondary to the distressing physical symptoms of hypersensitivity: this patient was initially classified as depressed, had no acute changes in psychological symptomatology on food exclusion/provocation, but her depression remitted completely after continued control of her physical symptoms by dietary exclusion. In contrast, there was positive evidence of significant psychiatric disturbance in all but 1 of the 18 patients whose belief that they had food allergy could not be confirmed. The psychiatric diagnoses in these patients are shown in table IV.

Table IV. Principal psychiatric diagnosis in patients falsely attributing somatic and psychological symptoms to food allergy [from ref. 117]

Depression	10
Neurasthenia	3
Hypochondriacal neurosis	1
Phobic state	1
Hysterical neurosis	1
Hysterical personality disorder	1
Not a psychiatric case	1

The patients presenting to our allergy clinic complaining of unconfirmable food allergy have also been compared to a random series of new patients referred to the psychiatric out-patients department of the same hospital [134]. This showed that the two groups were almost identical in terms of general characteristics and in the spectrum and severity of psychological symptoms. The only significant differences between the two were that the unconfirmable food allergy group contained a preponderance of professional people as opposed to a lower socio-economic grouping in the psychiatric out-patients, and that the allergy clinic patients scored lower for both the reported symptoms and outward manifestations of anxiety.

A limited follow-up of the patients with unconfirmable food allergy indicated an association between prognosis and persistence of their belief. When told that we considered we had excluded food allergy, 7 patients rapidly came to accept this advice, and 7 initially rejected it. There was a remission, or major improvement in the symptoms of 6 of the former. In the seventh, interstitial cystitis was considered responsible for many of her somatic symptoms. However, 1 patient, who improved initially and who had a hysterical personality disorder, presented at another hospital within a few weeks complaining of a completely new set of symptoms. Improvement in symptoms occurred apparently otherwise spontaneously in some patients; but in others, it followed acceptance of more direct treatment of hyperventilation, anxiety or depression. Symptoms tended to persist in patients who refused to accept that they did not have food allergies. However, 2 patients from this group later improved and came to eat the foods they had avoided previously. In 1 patient this followed antidepressant treatment and in the other, a change to an occupation he found less stressful. Examination of total psychiatric symptom scores on the initial

Clinical Interview Schedule did not support the hypothesis that acceptance/non-acceptance of advice regarding allergy, or failure to comply with investigations, were purely a result of the severity of the underlying psychiatric disorder.

Genesis of Pseudo-Allergy

It is apparent that a group of patients exist who mistakenly believe that they have food allergy. The natural history of this situation is that patients suffering from various other conditions first become convinced that they have hidden allergies without associating their symptoms with specific foods. Often individual foods are then 'identified' as responsible. Initially apparent food-symptom associations are coincidental or due to misinterpretation, but in some cases psychogenic reactions to foods then develop. As a result of these false beliefs the patients' physical and psychological health are put at further risk. Therefore we need to consider the origins of this syndrome, which we shall call pseudo-food allergy (PFA), and examine how it can be managed.

A number of factors seem relevant to how and why patients come to the mistaken conclusion that they have food allergy. There can be little doubt that the considerable publicity given to the subject in all branches of the popular media in the UK recently has been a major influence. On top of this, in our own area public meetings have been held by clinical ecologists and leaflets promoting their claims and services are on display in health-food stores. This publicity must have affected the degree to which potential patients have sought out further information and specialist consultation. In addition the dearth of objective data in the professional literature has left many non-specialist practitioners uncertain as to how to respond to their patients' enquiries.

11 of the 19 unconfirmable food allergy patients in our first study had received advice that they had food allergy from medical or paramedical personnel, who were rarely their family physician. Some had gone directly to 'fringe-medicine' practitioners, but others had turned to them only after feeling that the advice they had received from orthodox practitioners was inadequate or incorrect. 6 of the 19 were initially convinced that they had food allergy by reading *Not all in the Mind* [96] and many others had their convictions reinforced by it. We have seen more than 20 similar patients since completing this study and all have either been told that they have multiple food allergies at private clinics or have been convinced by popular books. In contrast, only 1 of the 20 comparison new psychiatric out-

patients had even heard of *Not all in the Mind* and even then she had not considered the possibility that she could have food allergy.

As we noted earlier, patients with 'unconfirmable allergy' differ in few formal respects from unselected new psychiatric out-patients. The former's rather higher social class may be relevant to their own, or their doctor's attribution of their symptoms; to their tendency to reject advice with which they do not agree and seek further opinions; and to their reading habits and application of 'self-help'. However, the attitudes of these patients to both their psychological and somatic symptoms are notable.

In a psychiatric study of patients with diarrhoea due to organic bowel diseases (other than IBS), *Goldberg* [65] found a 34% incidence of minor psychiatric disorder. He concluded that the bowel and psychiatric problems were independent and that the former were unlikely to be the cause of the latter in the group as a whole. Psychiatric symptoms were independent of the frequency of bowel symptoms. However, the frequency with which patients attended the clinic and the degree of distress experienced in response to abnormal bowel action were found to be related to the psychiatric state. A much higher incidence of psychiatric disorder (86%) was found using similar methods in our own study of patients with IBS [11]. Comparison of these results suggests that the psychological abnormalities are not the result of the bowel symptoms in the majority of IBS patients. It was notable that many IBS patients continued to complain bitterly of 'diarrhoea' when they had what others would consider a normal bowel action.

Similarly, many PFA patients have a very fixed view of ideal health frequently referring to how they 'should' function or feel. Any minor departure from this abstract ideal seems to cause them significant distress. Some of their 'complaints' would be taken by the generality of the population either as being within the range of normal function, or as acceptable and understandable responses to external events. Examples from our own patients include: somnolence after large meals, prolonged car driving, or chronic voluntary sleep restriction; and changes in bowel habit in response to major fluctuations in fibre/fluid intake, or after ingestion of intestinal irritants such as curries and chilli peppers.

Depressive neurosis is the commonest psychiatric diagnosis in PFA patients [117]. Depressed patients commonly present with somatic complaints [33, 99]. Many will deny mood disturbance, others will rationalize it as a response to their predicament. Some of these complaints may

Table V. Common physical symptoms in depression [derived from ref. 99, 177]

Tiredness, exhaustion, weakness, fatigability
Sleep disturbance, daytime drowsiness
Breathing difficulty, rapid breathing, dry mouth
Dizziness, tinnitus, blurred vision, impaired concentration
Headaches; chest pain, abdominal or generalized pain
Appetite disturbance, weight loss or gain
Excessive perspiration, salivation; constipation
Disturbed sexual function

be the somatic features of the depressive state itself (e.g. lethargy, paucity of thought and activity, sleep disturbance, etc.; table V), others related to fears that they have an underlying fatal disease, and some related to a reduced tolerance to normal bodily sensations. PFA patients are unusual in that they tend to present with predominantly psychological symptoms for which they seek an organic label. The true nature of these symptoms may be denied even when others would consider them an entirely justifiable response to external events. As a group they reject psychiatry, apparently considering that a 'psychological' explanation implies moral censure and that their symptoms are not real. Similar ignorance of mind-body relationships was demonstrated in a promotional leaflet from a local ecology clinic, which stated that use of the term psychosomatic is 'the crime of accusing patients of suffering imaginary complaints'.

As a result of their interpretation of the significance of psychiatric diagnoses these patients desperately seek a less threatening explanation. Most will refuse psychiatric referral and several of our patients have stopped medicines they have suspected (mistakenly) of having psychoactive properties. 2 refused antidepressants on the grounds that they could not cope with the implications should the treatment cure their symptoms. In contrast to many depressed patients who fear they have cancer, one of our pseudo-allergy patients declared that he would welcome this diagnosis but 'If I thought I was a case of clinical depression I would shoot myself'. A more general rejection of all orthodox medicine may be reflected by a propensity to consult 'fringe' practitioners: several of our patients tried other forms of alternative medicine either before or after suffering from 'food allergy'. 3 of the patients from our first study reported 'reactions' to virtually every medicine ever prescribed for them. 2 of these were openly hostile to the whole medical establishment.

In many patients the belief in food allergy may be considered as having the status of an *overvalued idea* [134]. This is supported by the persistence and tenacity with which it is held (for example, 2 of our patients who continued to insist they had a hidden food allergy despite being unable to identify any food-symptom associations on any protocol). The investment of considerable affect in the idea was demonstrated by the hostility with which many of our patients reacted to any attempt to challenge their belief. In some cases, comparison of case histories taken before and after specific exclusion reveals no actual change in symptom frequency, despite the patient's insistence that they are improved. Others, claiming relief as long as they stick to their diet, explain persistent symptoms by assuming that they have inadvertently broken their diet. However, recurrence of symptoms is often seen as evidence of yet another allergy and the need for further dietary restriction. The result of such sequential self-diagnosis is often a bizarre and dangerous diet: many of our patients have suffered severe weight loss as a result of severe calorie restriction, others have been at significant risk of vitamin deficiency states. Both we and our paediatrician colleagues at this hospital have seen children whose failure to thrive has been a direct result of dietary manipulation for presumed allergy. Every patient seen at our clinic over the last 4 years, who has believed themselves sensitive to more than one major food group (whether or not hypersensitivity has been confirmed subsequently) and who has been subjected to a formal dietary assessment has had a diet deficient in some essential nutrient.

Pseudo-allergy patients therefore do appear to have some distinguishing features. But what are the mechanisms by which their symptoms are produced? In a few of our cases some of the somatic symptoms have been produced by another organic disease process. This may be overlooked or improperly treated if the patient, or those he consults, attribute all the symptoms to one process. Many symptoms attributed to food allergy by these patients could be considered the common features and somatic concomitants of depressive illness (table V). Others may be explained by anxiety and associated sympathetic activity. Hyperventilation is certainly responsible for many of the symptoms in a significant proportion of the patients. Unfortunately we were not fully aware of the importance of the chronic hyperventilation syndrome (HVS, reviewed by *Lum* in this volume) when we commenced our studies, but in retrospect 11 of our 19 'unconfirmable allergy' patients had symptom complexes suggestive of HVS. The last 3 patients included in that study did have voluntary hyper-

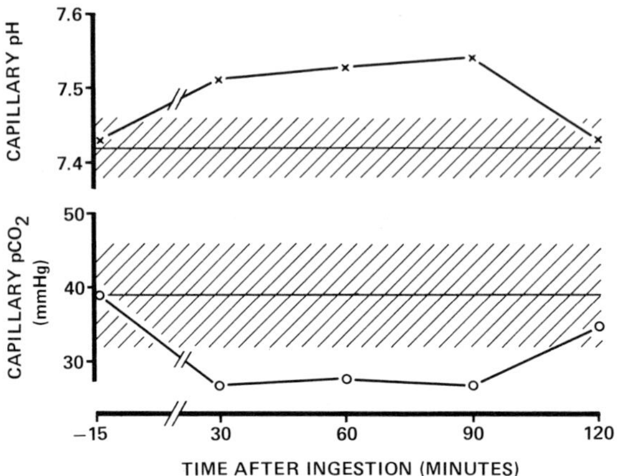

Fig. 2. Blood-gas changes on open wheat provocation in a patient complaining of multiple food allergies. Symptoms attributed to food included: tiredness, sleepiness, muscle weakness and spasms, back/neck and joint pains, aching all over, peripheral 'swelling', acroparasthesiae, blue hands, rapid pulse, closed-up throat, mood swings, irritability, crying spells, swollen eyes, disorientation, blurred vision and episodes of 'collapse'. Several produced within 2 min of open provocation and voluntary hyperventilation; inconsistent on DB provocation. Symptoms relieved by bag rebreathing and by 5% CO_2 in air.

ventilation tests, which reproduced several of their symptoms in 2 cases. In our subsequent experience we have found that HVS accounts for a significant proportion of the symptoms in about 60% of the 'food allergy' patients referred to us. Typical blood-gas changes following open wheat challenge, in a patient who believed she was wheat sensitive, and in whom voluntary hyperventilation reproduced all her symptoms are shown in figure 2.

How are symptoms associated with food? In some cases no consistent associations are observable, but coincidental changes are misattributed by the patient as a result of their overvalued idea. High suggestibility could explain how some patients become convinced they have food allergy simply on reading a book; the initial symptomatic improvement often observed on exclusion diets; repeated subjective reactions on open food reintroduction; and the high placebo response rates observed during double blind studies. The suggestive power of concentrated interest on dietary manipulation was demonstrated in our study of irritable bowel syndrome, in which almost 50% of patients, who had never previously considered themselves allergic, and in whom food hypersensitivity could not be confirmed subsequently, came to consider that specific foods were responsible for their symptoms at some time in the course of their investigation.

In the case of patients with HVS, the apprehension associated with ingesting a suspected food may be adequate to trigger an attack. Diaphragmatic splinting due to gastric distension may also result in meal-related changes in breathing pattern. Other potential mechanisms have not been adequately investigated in pseudo-allergy. Sleepiness is common after heavy meals and depressed patients, who tolerate any symptoms poorly and who already have a subclinical level of 'lethargy', may react with distress to further lowering of their feelings of energy by a normal degree of post-prandial torpor. Episodes described as depression or fatigue, as well as anxiety, can sometimes be related to neuroglycopaenia and sympathetic activity secondary to reactive hypoglycaemia [176]. These and other symptoms may occur in the several 'dumping syndromes'. We did have some evidence to incriminate early rapid rises in blood glucose and late hypoglycaemia in the generation of some of the symptoms in 1 of our pseudo-allergy patients with a long history of peptic ulceration. Unfortunately he then failed to co-operate with further investigations.

Management of Pseudo-Allergy

One could argue that the reasons why patients improve are immaterial as long as they feel better. It could be regarded as a satisfactory outcome if patients come to feel well after receiving a non-threatening explanation for their symptoms, or as a result of the placebo effect of treatment for supposed allergies. This may well occur in some cases. However, we have seen that the diagnosis of food allergy has very real dangers: it may affect adversely the prognosis of psychiatric disorders and coincidental physical illnesses and lead directly to new physical problems.

Many pseudo-allergy patients take diets which are positively harmful to their physical health. Weight loss due to total calorie deficit is common and mineral and vitamin deficiences are a real risk. An important aim in their management must be to prevent or correct this, whenever possible, by making sure they have a nutritionally adequate diet. In the presence of genuine allergy, or when patients refuse to accept its absence, suitable vitamin and mineral supplements must be provided. Particular attention should be paid to vitamin D and calcium requirements in the case of children and women of child-bearing age, as milk is one of the most frequently excluded foods and a vital source of these factors. The assistance of a properly trained dietician is invaluable in assessing and planning this aspect of the patient's management.

Properly performed, full dietary exclusion protocols are difficult and time consuming for both patient and physician. They also run the risk of further reinforcing the concept of food as a cause of the patient's symptoms. In the light of our earlier results we now consider that formal full investigation of allergy should only be undertaken in patients presenting with psychological and other non-atopic conditions if they persist in attributing symptoms to food after other avenues have been explored. However double blind provocations are sometimes useful in the course of other investigations to demonstrate the inconsistency of the reactions to the patient.

The initial assessment of patients attributing symptoms to foods will include a full allergological history, skin prick testing and a dietary history. The latter should include an assessment of nutritional intake. Attention should be given to the possibility of genuine anaphylactoid reactions, confusion regarding which can lead to multiple foods being blamed incorrectly. The presence of other organic conditions as a cause of at least some of the patient's symptoms must be borne in mind and appropriate investigations instituted when appropriate. A psychiatric diagnosis should not be made purely on the basis of exclusion of recognized organic conditions, but on the basis of positive features revealed by a careful psychiatric and social history and mental state examination.

Some pseudo-allergy patients will benefit from formal psychiatric treatment and this is much facilitated if the psychiatrist is seen as part of the team investigating 'allergy' and is involved at an early stage. We are fortunate in this regard in having an arrangement in which a liaison psychiatrist is attached to our medical unit. However, patients with less severe degrees of disturbance can often be managed without the direct involvement of a psychiatrist, particularly if adequate attention is given to the two most common underlying processes: hyperventilation syndrome and depressive illness.

We now perform a test of voluntary hyperventilation early in the course of the investigation of any patient with features suggestive of HVS. Not only does production of presenting symptoms provide a diagnosis, but it demonstrates their non-allergic basis to the patient, and, if combined with bag rebreathing, shows them a means of controlling their more frightening symptoms. Most patients derive comfort from realizing the chemical basis of their symptoms and that their doctor does not consider them to be imaginary. Some patients require no other therapy. Others, who would not previously accept treatment for the affective states leading to their hyperventilatory response, will subsequently do so. While it is not necessary in every case, in patients who are very confident of their allergies it is useful to perform an open food provocation with monitoring of blood gases, prior to the voluntary hyperventilation test.

Whether or not they also hyperventilate, patients presenting with pseudo-allergy are often depressed. A proportion of depressed patients respond to tricyclic antidepressants even when the depressive state is apparently secondary to other medical or social events. Somatic features such as early morning waking, diurnal variation in mood, appetite, energy and libido disturbances indicate a probable beneficial response to antidepressants. It is well worth a therapeutic trial of a tricyclic over a minimum period of 1 month, in any patient with persistent depressive features. Although initially rejecting 'psychological models of illness', many of these patients will accept this form of treatment if it is presented as part of a more general investigation and treatment package.

The subgroup of pseudo-allergy patients with hysterical and other personality disorders are particularly difficult to manage. Some persist in declaring they suffer from allergies. Others who initially appear to improve after accepting that they do not, rapidly develop new symptoms or new self-diagnoses for a recurrence of their old symptoms. Regrettably the false belief in food allergy can be very persistent once it has been established and a significant proportion of the whole pseudo-allergy patient group refuse to accept the evidence concerning the true nature of their symptoms. These patients will continue to be at risk of superimposing dietary deficiency diseases on top of their other problems. It would seem that prevention would be vastly preferable to this situation. This would be aided by a greater availability of properly trained specialists in allergy and by a wider dissemination of accurate information about allergic and hypersensitivity diseases.

References

1 Aas, K.: The diagnosis of hypersensitivity to ingested foods. Clin. Allergy *8:* 39 (1978).

2 Aitken, R.C.B.; Zealley, A.K.; Rosenthal, S.V.: Psychological and physiological measures of emotion in chronic asthmatic patients. J. psychosom. Res. *13:* 289 (1969).

3 Alvarez, W.C.: Food sensitivities and conditions that may be confused with it. Med. Clins N. Am. *12:* 1589 (1929).

4 Andreson, A.F.R.: Gastrointestinal manifestations of food allergy. Med. J. Rec. *122:* 271 (1925).

5 Anonymous clinical ecologist: BBC Radio, Manchester Broadcast (1983).

6 Ashkenazi, A.; Krasilowsky, D.; Levin, S.; Idar, D.; Kalian, M.; Or, A.; Ginat, Y.; Halperin B.: Immunologic reaction of psychotic patients to fractions of gluten. Am. J. Psychiat. *136:* 1306 (1979).

7 Basomba, A.; Pelaez, A.; Campos, A.; Villalmanzo, I.G.: Aspirin-sensitive asthma (Letter). J. Allergy clin. Immunol. *68:* 484 (1981).

8 Bassoe, P.: The auriculotemporal syndrome and other vasomotor disturbances about the head: 'auriculotemporal syndrome' complicating diseases of the parotid gland: angioneurotic edema of the brain. Med. Clins N. Am. *16:* 405 (1932).

9 Beall, J.G.: Food additives and hyperactivity in children. Congressional Record S19736 (1973).

10 Berg, T.; Bennich, H.; Johansson, S.G.O.: In vitro diagnosis of allergy. A comparison between provocation tests and the radioallergosorbent test. Int. Archs Allergy appl. Immun. *40:* 770 (1971).

11 Bentley, S.J.; Pearson, D.J.; Rix, K.J.B.: Food hypersensitivity in irritable bowel syndrome. Lancet *ii:* 295 (1983).

12 Ben-Zui, Z.; Spohn, W.A.; Young, S.H.; Kattan, S.H.: Hypnosis for exercise-induced asthma. Am. Rev. resp. Dis. *125:* 392 (1982).

13 Bernstein, M.; Day, J.H.; Welsh, A.: Double-blind food challenge in the diagnosis of food sensitivity in the adult. J. Allergy clin. Immunol. *70:* 205 (1982).

14 Blackley, C.H.: Experimental researches on the causes and nature of catarrhus aestivus (Bailliere, Tindall & Cox, London 1873).

15 Block, J.; Jennings, P.; Harvey, E.; Simpson, E.: Interaction between allergic potential and psychopathology in childhood asthma. Psychosom. Med. *26:* 307 (1964).

16 Block, K.J.; Walker, W.A.: Effect of locally induced anaphylaxis on the uptake of bystander antigen. J. Allergy clin. Immunol. *67:* 312 (1981).

17 Bock, S.A.: Food sensitivity: a critical review and practical approach. Am. J. Dis. Child. *134:* 973 (1980).

18 Bock, S.A.: The natural history of food sensitivity. J. Allergy clin. Immunol. *69:* 173 (1982).

19 Bock, S.A.; Lee, W.Y.; Remigio, L.; Holst, A.; May, C.D.: Appraisal of skin tests with food extracts for diagnosis of food hypersensitivity. Clin. Allergy *8:* 559 (1978).

20 Boushey, H.A.: Bronchial hyperreactivity to sulfur dioxide: physiologic and political implications. J. Allergy clin. Immunol. *69:* 335 (1982).

21 Brandstaeg, P.; Tolo, K.: Mucosal permeability enhanced by serum-derived antibodies. Nature, Lond. *266:* 262 (1977).

22 Bringel, R.: Allergi i centrala nervsystemet. Nord. Med. *14:* 521 (1937); quoted by Speer, 1970, in ref. 63.

23 Brown, M.; Gibney, M.; Husband, P.R.; Radcliffe, M.: Food allergy in polysymptomatic patients. Practitioner *225:* 1651 (1981).

24 Bryant, D.H.; Burns, M.W.; Lazarus, L.: The correlation between skin tests, bronchial provocation and the serum level of IgE specific for common allergens in patients with asthma. Clin. Allergy *5:* 145 (1975).

25 Chafee, F.H.; Settipane, G.A.: Asthma caused by FD and C approved dyes. J. Allergy *40:* 65 (1967).

26 Champion, R.H.; Roberts, S.O.E.; Carpenter, R.G.; Roger, J.H.: Urticaria and angio-edema. A review of 554 patients. Br. J. Derm. *81:* 588 (1969).
27 Chiu, J.T.: Improvement in aspirin-sensitive asthmatic subjects after rapid aspirin desensitization and aspirin maintenance treatment. J. Allergy clin. Immunol. *71:* 560 (1983).
28 Chua, Y.Y.; Bremner, K.; Lakdawalla, N.; Llobet, J.L.; Kokubu, H.L.; Orange, R.P.; Collins-Williams, C.: In vivo and in vitro correlates of food allergy. J. Allergy clin. Immunol. *58:* 300 (1976).
29 Committee on Provocative Food Testing. Ann. Allergy *31:* 375 (1973).
30 Cooke, R.A.; Van der Veer, A.: Human sensitization. J. Immun. *1:* 201 (1916).
31 Coombs, R.R.A.; Gell, P.G.H.: Classification of allergic reactions responsible for hypersensitivity and disease; in Gell, Coombs, Lachmann, Clinical aspects of immunology (Blackwell, Oxford 1975).
32 Cooper, B.: Epidemiology; in Wing, Schizophrenia: towards a new synthesis, pp. 31–51 (Academic Press, London, 1978).
33 Creed, F.H.; Murphy, E.: The relationship between physical and psychological symptoms; in Creed, Pfeffer, Medicine and psychiatry: a practical approach, pp. 62–63 (Pitman, London 1982).
34 Crook, W.G.; Harrison, W.E.; Crawford, S.E.; Emerson, B.S.: Systems manifestations due to allergy. Paediatrics *27:* 790 (1961).
35 Crowe, W.R.: Cerebral allergic oedema. J. Allergy *13:* 173 (1941/42).
36 Dean, G.; Hanniffy, L.; Stevens, F.; Temperley, I.; O'Broid, J.D.; Scott, J.; Cahalane, S.F.: Schizophrenia and coeliac disease. J. Ir. med. Ass. *68:* 545 (1975).
37 Delaney, J.C.: The diagnosis of aspirin idiosyncrasy by analgesic challenge. Clin. Allergy *6:* 177 (1976).
38 Denman, A.M.: The relevance of immunopathology to research into schizophrenia; in Hemmings, Biochemistry of schizophrenia and addiction, pp. 97–109 (MTP Press, Lancaster 1980).
39 Dickey, L.D.: Clinical ecology (Thomas, Springfield 1976).
40 Doeglas, H.M.G.: Reactions to aspirin and food additives in patients with chronic urticaria, including the physical urticarias. Br. J. Derm. *93:* 135 (1975).
41 Dohan, F.C.: Wartime changes in hospital admissions for schizophrenia. Acta psychiat. scand. *42:* 1 (1966).
42 Dohan, F.C.: Cereals and schizophrenia. Data and hypothesis. Acta psychiat. scand. *42:* 125 (1966).
43 Dohan, F.C.: The possible pathogenic effect of cereal grains in schizophrenia. Celiac disease as a model. Acta neurol., Napoli *31:* 195 (1976).
44 Dohan, F.C.: Schizophrenia and neuroactive peptides from food (Letter). Lancet *i:* 1031 (1979).
45 Dohan, F.C.; Martin, L.; Grasberger, J.C.; Boehme, D.; Cottrell, J.C.: Antibodies to wheat gliadin in blood of psychiatric patients: possible role of emotional factors. Biol. Psychiat. *5:* 127 (1972).
46 Dohan, F.C.; Grasberger, J.C.; Lowell, F.M.; Johnston, J.P.; H.T.; Arbegast, A.W.: Relapsed schizophrenics: more rapid improvement on a milk and cereal-free diet. Br. J. Psychiat. *115:* 595 (1969).
47 Dohan, F.C.; Grasberger, J.C.: Relapsed schizophrenics: earlier discharge from the hospital after cereal-free, milk-free diet. Am. J. Psychiat. *130:* 685 (1973).

48 Duke, W.W.: Food allergy as a cause of bladder pain. Archs intern. Med. *29:* 178 (1922).
49 Duke, W.W.: Specific tests in the diagnosis of allergy. Archs intern. Med. *32:* 298 (1923).
50 Edgell, P.G.: Psychiatric approach to the treatment of bronchial asthma. Mod. Treat. *3:* 900 (1966).
51 Editorial: Feingold's regimen for hyperkinesis. Lancet *ii:* 617 (1979).
52 Eyerman, C.H.: Allergic headache. J. Allergy *11:* 106 (1931).
53 Executive Committee of the American Academy of Allergy. American Academy of Allergy: Position statements – controversial techniques. J. Allergy clin. Immunol. *67:* 333 (1981).
54 Falliers, C.J.: Psychosomatic study and treatment of children. Pediat. Clins N. Am. *16:* 271 (1969).
55 Feingold, B.: Introduction to clinical allergy (Thomas, Springfield 1973).
56 Feingold, B.: Why is your child hyperactive? (Random House, New York 1975).
57 Feingold, B.; German, D.F.; Braham, R.M.; Simmers, E.: Adverse reactions to food additives. Annual Convention of the American Medical Association, New York 1973.
58 Finn, R.; Cohen, N.H.: Food allergy: fact or fiction? Lancet *i:* 426 (1978).
59 Frank, N.R.; Amdur, M.O.; Worcester, J.; Whittenberger, J.C.: Effects of acute controlled SO_2 on respiratory mechanics in healthy male adults. J. appl. Physiol. *17:* 252 (1962).
60 Freedman, B.J.: Asthma induced by sulphur dioxide, benzoate and tartrazine in orange drinks. Clin. Allergy *7:* 407 (1977).
61 Freeman, E.; Feingold, B.; Schlesinger, K.; Gorman, F.: Psychological variables in allergic disorders: a review. Psychosom. Med. *26:* 543 (1964).
62 French, T.N.; Alexander, F.: Psychogenic factors in bronchial asthma. Psychsom. Med. Monogr. (National Research Council, Washington 1947).
63 Gibson, A.; Clancy, R.: Management of chronic idiopathic urticaria by the identification and exclusion of dietary factors. Clin. Allergy *10:* 699 (1980).
64 Glaisher, I.L.: Allergy and psychosis. Can. med. Ass. J. *111:* 1048 (1974).
65 Goldberg, D.P.: A psychiatric study of patients with diseases of the small intestine. Gut *11:* 549 (1970).
66 Graham, P.J.; Rutter, M.L.; Yule, W.; Pless, I.B.: Childhood asthma: a psychosomatic disorder? Some epidemiological considerations. Br. J. prev. soc. Med. *21:* 78 (1967).
67 Graham, D.T.; Wolf, S.; Wolf, H.G.: Changes in tissue sensitivity associated with varying life situations and emotions; their relevance to allergy. J. Allergy *21:* 478 (1950).
68 Hargreave, F.E.; Ryan, G.; Thomson, N.C.; O'Byrne, P.M.; Latimer, K.; Dolovich, J.: Bronchial responsiveness to histamine or metacholine in asthma: measurement and clinical significance. J. Allergy clin. Immunol. *68:* 347 (1981).
69 Harley, J.P.; Ray, R.S.; Tomas, L.; Eichman, P.L.; Mathews, C.G.; Chun, R.; Cleeland, C.S.; Transman, E.: Hyperkinesis and food additives: testing the Feingold hypothesis. Pediatrics *61:* 816 (1978).
70 Hekkens, W.T.J.M.: Antibodies to gliadin in serum of normals, coeliac patients and schizophrenics; in Hemmings, Hemmings, The biological basis of schizophrenia, pp. 259–261 (MTP Press, Lancaster 1978).
71 Hekkens, W.T.J.M.; Schipperyn, A.J.M.; Freed, D.L.J.: Antibodies to wheat proteins in schizophrenia: relationship of coincidence? In Hemmings, Biochemistry of schizophrenia and addiction, pp. 125–133 (MTP Press, Lancaster 1980).

72 Hoobler, B.R.: Some early symptoms suggesting protein sensitization in infancy. Am. J. Dis. Child. *12:* 129 (1916).

73 Huggins, K.G.; Brostoff, J.: Local production of specific IgE antibodies in allergic rhinitis patients with negative skin tests. Lancet *ii:* 148 (1975).

74 Hutinel, P.: Intolérance pour le lait et anaphlaxie chez les nourrissons. Clinique *3:* 227 (1908).

75 Jackson, P.G.; Lessof, M.H.; Baker, B.W.R.; Ferret, J.; MacDonald, D.M.: Intestinal permeability in patients with eczema and food allergy. Lancet *i:* 1285 (1981).

76 Jenner, A.: Conference on Trends in Biological Psychiatry, covered by Schizophrenia Association of Great Britain, Bedford College, London. Psychiat. Top. *4:* 8 (1983).

77 Kailin, E.W.; Collier, R.: 'Relieving' therapy for antigen exposure. J. Am. med. Ass. *217:* 78 (1971).

78 Kennedy, F.: Cerebral symptoms induced by angioneurotic oedema. Archs Neurol. Psychiat. *15:* 28 (1926).

79 Kennedy, F.: Certain nervous complications following use of therapeutic and prophylactic sera. J. Am. med. Ass. *177:* 555 (1929).

80 Kennedy, F.: Allergy and its effect on the central nervous system. Archs Neurol. *39:* 1361 (1938).

81 King, D.S.: Can allergic exposure provoke psychological symptoms? A double-blind test. Biol. Psychiat. *16:* 3 (1981).

82 Kinnell, H.G.; Kirkwood, E.; Lewis, C.: Food antibodies in schizophrenia. Psychol. Med. *12:* 85 (1982).

83 Koenig, J.Q.; Pierson, W.E.; Frank, R.: Acute effects of inhaled SO_2 plus NACI droplet aerosol on pulmonary function in asthmatic adolescents. Environ. Res. *22:* 14 (1980).

84 Koenig, J.Q.; Pierson, W.E.; Horicke, M.; Frank, R.: Effects of SO_2 plus NaCl aerosol combined with moderate exercise on pulmonary function in asthmatic adolescents. Environ. Res. *25:* 340 (1981).

85 Koenig, J.Q.; Pierson, W.E.; Horike, M.; Frank, R.: Bronchoconstrictor responses to sulfur dioxide or sulfur dioxide plus sodium chloride droplets in allergic, nonasthmatic adolescents. J. Allergy clin. Immunol. *69:* 339 (1982).

86 Kushe, J.: Oxidative deamination of biogenic amines by intestinal amine-oxydases: histamine is specially inactivated by diamine oxidase. Physiol. Chem. Phys. *356:* 1485 (1975).

87 Lee, C.H.: A new test for diagnosis and treatment of food allergies. Buchanan med. Bull. *25:* 9 (1961).

88 Lehman, C.W.: A double-blind study of sublingual provocative food testing: a study of its efficacy. Ann. Allergy *45:* 144 (1980).

89 Leonard, G.: Behavioural manifestations of allergic children. Ann. Allergy *24:* 248 (1966).

90 Lessof, M.H.: Food intolerance and allergy – a review. Q. Jl Med. *52:* 111 (1983).

91 Lessof, M.H.; Wraith, D.G.; Merrett, T.G.; Merrett, J.; Buisseret, P.D.: Food allergy and intolerance in 100 patients. Local and systemic effects. Q. Jl Med. *49:* 259 (1980).

92 Levy, D.L.; Weinreb, H.J.: Wheat-gluten schizophrenia findings (Letter). Science *194:* 448 (1976).

93 Lindhall, K.M.: The histamine methylating system in liver. Acta physiol. scand. *49:* 114 (1960).

94 Lockey, S.D.: Reactions to hidden agents in foods, beverages and drugs. Ann. Allergy *29:* 461 (1971).
95 Logan, W.P.D.: Mortality in the London fog incident. Lancet *i:* 336 (1953).
96 MacKarness, R.: Not all in the mind (Pan Books, London 1976).
97 Marley, E.; Thomas, D.V.: Histamine and its metabolites in cat portal venous blood and intestine after duodenal instillation of histamine. J. Physiol. *263:* 273 (1976).
98 Mattes, J.A.; Gittelman, R.: Effects of artificial food colourings in children with hyperactive symptoms. Archs gen. Psychiat. *38:* 714 (1981).
99 Mathew, R.J.; Weinman, M.L.; Mirabi, M.: Physical symptoms of depression. Br. J. Psychiat. *139:* 293 (1981).
100 May, C.D.: Objective clinical and laboratory studies of immediate hypersensitivity reactions to foods in asthmatic children. J. Allergy clin. Immunol. *58:* 500 (1976).
101 May, C.D.: Food allergy: lessons from the past. J. Allergy clin. Immunol. *69:* 255 (1982).
102 McDonald, J.R.; Mathison, D.A.; Stevenson, D.E.: Aspirin intolerance in asthma. Detection by oral challenge. J. Allergy clin. Immunol. *50:* 198 (1972).
103 McGovern, J.P.; Knight, J.A.: Allergy and human emotions (Thomas, Springfield 1967).
104 McGuffin, P.; Gardiner, P.; Swinburne, L.M.: Schizophrenia, celiac disease and antibodies to foods. Biol. Psychiat. *16:* 281 (1981).
105 Michaelsson, G.; Juhlin, L.: Urticaria induced by preservatives and dye additives in food and drugs. Br. J. Derm. *88:* 535 (1973).
106 Moneret-Vautrin, D.A.: Food pseudo-allergy; in Pepys, Edwards, The mast cell (Pitman Medical, London 1979).
107 Moneret-Vautrin, D.A.: False food allergies: non-specific reactions to foodstuffs; in Lessof, Clinical reactions to food, pp. 135–153 (Wiley, Chichester 1983).
108 Morris, D.L.: Use of sublingual antigen in diagnosis and treatment of food allergy. Ann. Allergy *27:* 289 (1971).
109 Nadel, J.A.; Salem, H.; Tamplin, B.; Tokiva, Y.: Mechanism of broncho-constriction during inhalation of sulphur dioxide, J. appl. Physiol. *20:* 164 (1965).
110 National Advisory Committee on Hyperkinesis and Food Additives: Report to the Nutrition Foundation (Nutrition Foundation, 1975).
111 National Institutes of Health consensus development conference statement: defined diets and childhood hyperactivity. Am. J. clin. Nutr. *37:* 161 (1983).
112 Neuhans, E.C.: A personality study of asthmatic and cardiac children. Psychosom. Med. *20:* 181 (1958).
113 Osborne, M.; Crayton, J.D.; Javaid, J.; Davies, J.M.: Lack of effect of a gluten-free diet on neuroleptic blood levels in schizophrenic patients. Biol. Psychiat. *17:* 627 (1982).
114 Oswald, N.C.; Waller, R.E.; Drinkwater, J.: Relationship between breathlessness and anxiety in asthma and bronchitis: a comparative study. Br. med. J. *ii:* 14 (1970).
115 Pardee, I.: Two cases demonstrating allergic reactions in the nervous system. J. nerv. ment. Dis. *88:* 89 (1938).
116 Paton, W.D.M.: The release of histamine. Prog. Allergy, vol. 5, p. 70 (Karger, Basel 1958).
117 Pearson, D.J.; Rix, K.J.B.; Bentley, S.J.: Food allergy: How much in the mind? Lancet *i:* 1259 (1983).
118 Pleskow, W.W.; Stevenson, D.D.; Mathison, D.A.; Simon, R.A.; Schatz, M.; Zeiger, R.S.: Aspirin desensitisation in aspirin-sensitive asthmatic patients: clinical

manifestations and characterisation of the refractory period. J. Allergy clin. Immunol. *63:* 11 (1982).
119 Potkin, S.G.; Weinberger, D.; Kleinman, J.; Nasrallah, H.; Luchins, D.; Bigelow, L.; Lianoila, M.; Fischer, D.H.; Bjornsson, T.D.; Garman, J.; Gillin, J.C.; Wyatt, R.J.: Wheat gluten challenge in schizophrenic patients. Am. J. Psychiat. *138:* 1208 (1981).
120 Prenner, B.M.; Stevens, J.J.: Anaphylaxis after ingestion of sodium bisulphite. Ann. Allergy *37:* 180 (1976).
121 Quevauvilles, A.; N'Guyen, Van Hoa: L'histamine dans quelques produits alimentaires d'origine occidentale ou extrême-orientale. Bull. Soc. scient. Hyg. aliment. *53:* 284 (1965).
122 Rachelefsky, G.S.; Coulson, A.; Siegel, S.C.; Steim, E.R.: Aspirin intolerance in chronic childhood asthma: detection by oral challenge. Pediatrics *56:* 443 (1975).
123 Randolph, T.G.: Descriptive features of food addictions, addictive eating and drinking. Q. Jl Stud. Alcohol *23:* 7 (1956).
124 Randolph, T.G.: Historical development of clinical ecology; in Dickey, Clinical ecology, pp. 9–17 (Thomas, Springfield 1976).
125 Randolph, T.G.: Adaption to specific environmental exposure and enhanced by individual susceptibility; in Dickey, Clinical ecology, pp. 46–66 (Thomas, Springfield 1976).
126 Randolph, T.G.: Hospital comprehensive environmental control programm; in Dickey, Clinical ecology, pp. 70–85 (Thomas, Springfield 1976).
127 Randolph, T.G.: Stimulatory and withdrawal levels and the alternations of allergic manifestations; in Dickey, Clinical ecology, pp. 156–175 (Thomas, Springfield 1976).
128 Randolph, T.G.; Moss, P.W.: Allergies: your hidden enemy. How the new science of clinical ecology is unravelling the causes of mental and physical illness. (Turnstone Press, Wellingborough 1981).
129 Rapp. D.J.: Double-blind confirmation and treatment of milk sensitivity. Med. J. Aust. *i:* 571 (1978).
130 Rinkel, H.J.: Food allergy. The role of food allergy in internal medicine. Ann. Allergy *2:* 115 (1944).
131 Rinkel, H.J.: The management of clinical allergy. II. Etiologic factors and skin titration. Archs Otolar. *77:* 42 (1963).
132 Rinkel, H.J.; Lee, C.H.; Brown, D.W.; Willougby, J.W.; Williams, J.M.: The diagnosis of food allergy. Archs Otolar. *79:* 71 (1964).
133 Rix, K.J.B.; Ditchfield, J.; Freed, D.L.T.; Goldberg, D.P.; Hillier, V.; Merrett, T.J.: Food antibodies in acute psychoses (in preparation, 1984).
134 Rix, K.J.B.; Bearson, D.J.; Bentley, S.J.: A psychiatric study of patients with supposed food allergy. Br. J. Psychiat. *145:* 126 (1984).
135 Ros, A.M.; Juhlin, L.; Michaelsson, G.: A follow-up study of patients with recurrent urticaria and hypersensitivity to aspirin, benzoates and azo dyes. Br. J. Derm. *95:* 19 (1976).
136 Rowe, A.H.: Food allergy: its manifestations, diagnosis and treatment. J. Am. med. Ass. *91:* 1623 (1928).
137 Rowe, A.H.: Food allergy. Its manifestations, diagnosis and treatment, with a general discussion of bronchial asthma (Bailliere, Tindal & Cox, London 1931).
138 Samter, M.; Beers, R.F.: Concerning the nature of intolerance to aspirin. J. Allergy *40:* 281 (1967).

139 Schachter, M.: Histamine release and the angio-oedema type of reaction; in Wolstenholme, O'Connor, Histamine. Ciba Foundation Symposium (Churchill, London 1956).
140 Schachter, M.; Talesnik, J.: The release of histamine by egg-white in non-sensitized animals. J. Physiol., Lond. *118:* 258 (1958).
141 Schartz, H.J.: Sensitivity to ingested meta-bisulphite: variations in clinical presentation. J. Allergy clin. Immunol. *71:* 487 (1983).
142 Schloss, O.M.: A case of allergy to common foods. Am. J. Dis. Child. *3:* 341 (1912).
143 Schloss, O.M.: Allergy in infants and children. Am. J. Dis. Child. *19:* 433 (1920).
144 Schlumberger, H.D.: Drug-induced pseudo-allergic syndrome as exemplified by acetylsalicyclic acid intolerance; in Dukor, Kallas, Schlumberger, West, Pseudo-allergic reactions (Karger, Basel 1980).
145 Selye, H.: The physiology and pathology of exposure to stress (Acta, Montreal 1950).
146 Sheppard, D.; Wong, W.S.; Uehara, C.F.; Nadel, J.A.; Boushey, H.A.: Lower threshold and greater bronchomotor responsiveness of asthmatic subjects to sulphur dioxide. Am. Res. resp. Dis. *122:* 873 (1980).
147 Singh, M.M.; Kay, S.R.: Wheat gluten as a pathogenic factor in schizophrenia. Science *191:* 401 (1976).
148 Smith, J.M.: Wheat-gluten schizophrenia findings (Letter). Science *194:* 448 (1976).
149 Speer, F.: The allergic tension-fatigue syndrome; in Allergy of the nervous system (Thomas, Springfield 1970).
150 Staffiere, D.; Dentolia, L.; Levit, L.: Hemiplegia and allergic symptoms following ingestion of certain foods. Ann. Allergy. *10:* 38 (1952).
151 Stenius, B.S.M.; Lemola, M.: Hypersensitivity to acetylsalicytic acid (ASA) and tartrazine in patients with asthma. Clin. Allergy *6:* 119 (1976).
152 Stevens, F.M.; Lloyd, R.S.; Gerachty, S.M.J.; Reynolds, M.T.G.; Sarsfield, M.J.; McNicholl, B.; Fottrell, P.F.; Wright, R.; McCarthy, C.F.: Schizophrenia and coeliac disease – the nature of the relationship. Psychol. Med. *7:* 259 (1977).
153 Stevenson, D.D.; Mathison, D.A.: Aero-allergen inhalation challenge in aspirin-intolerant asthmatic patients. J. Allergy clin. Immunol. *55:* 127 (1975).
154 Stevenson, D.D.; Simon, R.A.; Mathison, D.H.: Aspirin-sensitive asthma: desensitisation after positive oral aspirin challenge. J. Allergy clin. Immunol. *66:* 82 (1980).
155 Stevenson, D.D.; Simon, R.A.: Sensitivity to ingested metabisulphites in asthmatic subjects. J. Allergy clin. Immunol. *68:* 26 (1981).
156 Storms, L.H.; Clopton, J.M.; Wright, C.: Effects of gluten on schizophrenics. Archs gen. Psychiat. *39:* 323 (1982).
157 Swanson, J.M.; Kinsbourne, M.: Food dyes impair performance of hyperactive children on a laboratory learning test. Science *207:* 1485 (1980).
158 Szentivanyi, A.: The beta adrenergic theory of atopic abnormality in bronchial asthma. J. Allergy *42:* 203 (1968).
159 Szentivanyi, A.; Fishel, C.W.: The beta-adrenergic theory and cyclic AMP mediated control mechanisms in human asthma; in Weiss, Segal, Bronchial asthma mechanisms and therapeutics (Little Brown, Boston 1976).
160 Tarlo, S.M.; Broder, I.: Tartrazine and benzoate challenge and dietary avoidance in chronic asthma. Clin. Allergy *12:* 303 (1982).
161 Taylor, E.: Annotation: food additives, allergy and hyperkinesis. J. Child Psychol. Psychiat. *20:* 353 (1979).

162 Turnbull, J.A.: Food allergies in connection with arthritis. Boston med. surg. J. *191:* 438 (1924).
163 Vaughan, V.C.: Emotional undertones in eczema in children. J. Asthma Res. *3:* 193 (1966).
164 Vaughan, W.T.; Hawke, I.K.: Angioneurotic oedema with some unusual manifestations. J. Allergy *2:* 125 (1931).
165 Vedanthan, P.K.; Menon, M.M.; Bell, T.D.; Bergin, D.: Aspirin and tartrazine oral challenge: incidence of adverse response in chronic childhood asthma. J. Allergy clin. Immunol. *60:* 8 (1977).
166 Ward, J.F.: Protein sensitization as a possible cause of epilepsy and cancer. N.Y. med. J. *115:* 592 (1922).
167 Warner, J.O.: The problems of diet in food intolerance and pseudo-intolerance. British Society for Immunology Food Allergy Workshop, 1983.
168 Weiss, B.; Williams, J.H.; Marjen, S.; et al.: Behavioural responses to artificial food colours. Science *207:* 1487 (1980).
169 Weiss, J.H.: Mood states associated with asthma in children. J. psychosom. Res. *10:* 267 (1966).
170 Wendel, E.: New evidence on food additives and hyperkenesis. Am. J. Dis. Child. *134:* 1122 (1980).
171 Wide, L.; Bennich, H.; Johansson, S.G.O.: Diagnosis of allergy by an in vitro test for allergic antibodies. Lancet *ii:* 1105 (1967).
172 Williams, J.I.; Cram, D.M.; Tausig, F.T.; Webster, E.: Relative effects of drugs and diet on hyperactive behaviours – an experimental study. Pediatrics *61:* 811 (1978).
173 Wittkower, E.: Studies on hay-fever patients. J. ment. Sci. *84:* 352 (1938).
174 Zeidberg, L.D.; Prindle, R.A.; Landau, E.: The Nashville air pollution study. I. Sulfur dioxide and bronchial asthma. Am. Rev. resp. Dis. *84:* 489 (1961).
175 Zeiss, C.R.; Lockey, R.F.: Refractory period to aspirin in a patient with aspirin-induced asthma. J. Allergy clin. Immunol. *57:* 440 (1976).
176 Hale, F.; Margen, S.; Rabak, D.: Post-prandial hypoglycaemia and 'psychological' symptoms. Biol. Psychiat. *17:* 125 (1981).
177 Beck, A.T.: Depression: clinical, experimental and theoretical aspects (Staples Press, London 1967).

David J. Pearson, PhD, MRCP, Department of Medicine, University Hospital of South Manchester, West Didsbury, Manchester M20 8LR (England)

PAR. Pseudo-Allergic Reactions. Involvement of Drugs and Chemicals, vol. 4, pp. 106–119 (Karger, Basel 1985)

Hyperventilation and Pseudo-Allergic Reactions[1]

L.C. Lum

Papworth and Addenbrooke's Hospitals, Cambridge, England

Introduction

Hyperventilation was described by *Darwin* [1] as an integral part of the reaction to perceived danger, a concept subsequently elaborated by *Cannon* [2] in describing the 'fight or flight' reaction and the physiological changes which prepare the body for defensive or offensive action. While these authors recognized its value in the reaction to danger, they were unaware of the ill results of inappropriate overbreathing.

The relevance of hyperventilation to allergic reactions is hardly apparent at first sight. Some concrete examples may serve as an introduction. Consider allergy to isocyanates, substances commonly used in the production of various plastic foams and in some paints. On exposure, susceptible persons may become sensitized and develop asthma. As medical adviser to a manufacturer using them, I was frequently called to examine personnel taken ill following spillage or other accidental exposure to higher than normal concentrations. Almost invariably complaints involved dizziness, faintness or collapse, often headache, oppression of the breathing, general malaise or nausea. These, however, are some of the commoner symptoms of acute hyperventilation, not of reaction to isocyanates. Even more significant, similar complaints were likely to follow

[1] *Physiological Terms.* Hyperventilation: Breathing in excess of body needs. – Carbon dioxide (CO_2): The gaseous end product of body metabolism. – Hypocapnoea or hypocarbia: Low value of carbon dioxide in the arterial blood (expressed as partial pressure of carbon dioxide in millimetres of mercury – arterial P_{CO_2} mm Hg). – Hypoxia: Low value of oxygen in blood and tissues. – Cerebral hypoxia: Insufficient oxygen supply for normal brain function. – Respiratory alkalosis: Occurs when alveolar P_{CO_2} is lowered by excessive ventilation. Chronic respiratory alkalosis is present when the P_{CO_2} remains significantly below 35 mm Hg.

inhalation of *any* vapours from solvents some of which had no known toxic action. The workforce, conditioned to working in a potentially toxic environment, reacted with alarm and hyperventilation to any suspicion of toxic exposure. Similar complaints can follow any television programme on asbestosis – at present, very much in the public eye.

Following an address to a meeting of food intolerance sufferers, more than 50% of the audience recognized that many of their presumed 'intolerance' symptoms tallied with those of overbreathing. Moreover, two, who had considered themselves to be allergic to the floor polish of the meeting room, identified their symptoms with those of hyperventilation, which was always triggered by smelling the polish. Voluntary overbreathing can produce similar symptoms.

Some asthmatics develop tremors and tachycardia following salbutamol inhalations and are regarded as sensitive to this agent. In this case, the relief of spasm, by allowing unobstructed respiration, permits overbreathing (to which asthmatics are prone). The tremors and tachycardia can usually be abolished by teaching patients not to overbreathe after such inhalations; thereafter, they are able to use salbutamol without ill effect. Supposed hypersensitivity to dental anaesthetics may occur in a similar way. Phobic reactions to hypodermic injections are common, producing hyperventilation and collapse. Recently, on trying to take a blood sample from a man, he began to overbreathe, collapsed to the floor, became rigid, and made jactitating movements. He remained stuporose for 1.5 h.

Examples can be elaborated *ad nauseam*. Recent publicity in England regarding 'total allergy' revealed that the symptoms of the latter were similar to those of hyperventilation. In several cases seen by the author, the symptoms could be initiated by hyperventilation and abolished by rebreathing from a *plastic* bag, – despite the fact that they were said to be sensitive to petrochemicals! A psychological reaction, with overbreathing, to a situation perceived as harmful, caused the symptoms.

Table I, compiled from the symptoms observed in a personal study of over 2,300 patients, illustrates the range and complexity of physiological disturbances encountered in chronic habitual hyperventilation.

The common pathway to this plethora of disturbances is the nervous system. Thus, in considering the physiological mechanisms involved, one must review the action of carbon dioxide on that system. Overbreathing discharges excessive amounts of carbon dioxide from the body, thus lowering the level of that gas in the arterial blood (hypocarbia). This affects primarily the brain and nervous system, since the carbon dioxide molecule

Table I. Symptoms commonly associated with hyperventilation states

Cardiac Palpitations, missed beats, tachycardia, 'angina', atypical chest pain, dull precordial or lower costal ache, vasomotor instability
Neurological Dizziness, faintness, visual disturbance, migrainous headache, numbness, paraesthesiae of limbs, face or elsewhere, intolerance of bright lights or loud noise
Respiratory Irritable cough, 'asthma', tight chest, excessive sighing or yawning
Gastro-intestinal Dysphagia, dry throat, flatulence and belching, aerophagy, upper abdominal distress, globus
Muscular Cramps, diffuse or localised myalgia, tremors or coarse twitches, rarely tetany
Psychic Tension, anxiety, 'unreal' feelings, depersonalisation, hallucination, fear of insanity, panic attacks, fear of sudden death, phobic states, agoraphobia
General Weakness, exhaustion, lack of concentration and memory, sleep disturbance, nightmares, emotional sweating (axillae and palms)

modulates the activity of most components of that system. Hence symptoms may be produced in any part of the body. Particularly disturbing are alterations in brain function, such as impaired mentation, diminished cortical inhibitory control, panic attacks, phobias, agoraphobia, depersonalisation, even hallucinations, and fear of madness. In order to understand the mechanisms involved, it is necessary to review the complex interrelationships between breathing disturbances, carbon dioxide, and the function of the brain and nervous system.

Breathing Disorder

Christie [3] in 1935 noted that the breathing pattern of patients thought to be 'neurotic' was so characteristic that he could make the diagnosis of 'neurosis' simply by inspection of the spirometer tracing, without reference to any other clinical data (fig. 1). A similar relationship had been observed by *du Laurens* [4] – without the benefit of instrumentation – in

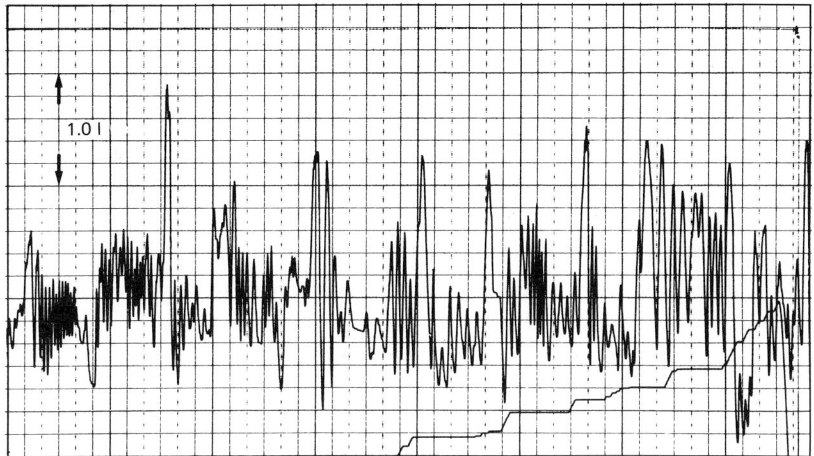

Fig. 1. Grossly abnormal spirogram in severe hyperventilator. Note frequent large sighing respirations, and great variation in amplitude and frequency of breaths.

1595! *Christie* [3] did not record P_{CO_2} changes but we now know that such breathing results in abrupt variations in P_{CO_2} of sufficient severity to cause symptoms via the physiological mechanisms to be described. Moreover, once the P_{CO_2} has fallen, it reverts only slowly to normal, as in the example shown in figure 3.

On occasions, the symptoms may be so alarming that hyperventilation escalates into a vicious cycle which eventually results in tetany or coma. Such attacks are relatively uncommon (less than 1% of my patients) but, regrettably, are the only manifestation of hyperventilation mentioned in current English texts. They are usually regarded as hysterical.

The breathing is characteristically fast, often 20–30 breaths/min, occasionally much higher. In extremely severe attacks, it may approach or exceed 60. There are wide variations in rate, rhythm and tidal volume. Sighing respirations are common, and when frequent are highly suggestive of the diagnosis (fig. 1). The breathing is almost entirely thoracic, with little, if any, apparent diaphragmatic excursion. Patients almost invariably have very poor control of their breathing.

Haldane and Poulton [5] were among the first to describe the effects of acute overbreathing in humans. In 1908 they alarmed the Physiological Society of London when *Poulton,* demonstrating overbreathing, became so profoundly collapsed, that the learned audience thought he had died and some 'had to retire hastily' [5]. Recognition that lesser, but still very severe, symptoms can be produced, came much later. *White and Hahn* [6] and *Kerr* et al. [7] first showed that the somatic manifestations of 'neurosis' or 'non-organic' illness were mediated by hyperventilation, and attributed them to respiratory alkalosis. Their papers were followed, in the ensuing decades, by many other papers implicating overbreathing as the physiological basis of psychosomatic symptoms [8–12]. A comprehensive review has been published by *Magarian* [13].

These, however, made little impact among the post-war plethora of advances in medical technology and pharmacology. In the same period, increasing specialization further orientated physicians towards disease processes rather than sick patients. Hence the concept of 'non-organic disease' became synonymous with 'neurosis' and served to relegate illness with no detectable organic lesion to the still nebulous world of psychiatric theory. The situation has now been reached where the vast majority of medical graduates and practising physicians are quite unaware of the existence, even less the variety, of syndromes whose basis is *chronic habitual hyperventilation* [13]. It is interesting to note that *Cannon* [2], in 1928, was deploring the reluctance of physicians to concern themselves with illness which did not have demonstrable pathology. One general physician found that cases exhibiting this symptomatology constituted 40.2% of referrals to his general medical clinic [14] and yet did not consider hyperventilation as a possible cause.He called them all anxiety states and considered that reassurance was sufficient treatment.

Lewis [10] described the symptoms as a 'welter of unpleasant bodily sensations'. The present writer would add 'welter of unpleasant bodily and mental sensations, with frequent phobias, fear of death, madness, or both' (table I). It is usual for sufferers to experience complaints related to several systems, but many symptoms will not be volunteered unless specifically enquired for, the patient concentrating either on those presently most worrying and often concealing those which he suspects will be regarded as neurotic or imaginary. On the other hand, patients will often recognize themselves when confronted with a list such as table I.

Overbreathing is a perfectly normal reaction to stress of any sort. Some explanation is needed as to how a normal reaction can produce a disabling illness. Firstly, habitual overbreathing may keep the Pa_{CO_2} near the symptomatic threshold so that minor stress can readily lower it to symptomatic levels. Secondly, the responsiveness of the breathing varies enormously from individual to individual. Quite apart from respiratory need, breathing is affected also by a very wide variety of stimuli, both from bodily sensations and from higher centres in the brain. Almost any change in environment will provoke a change in respiration, e.g. breath-holding followed by rapid breathing, gasping, or sighing. This respiratory reaction is probably the most immediate response to any stimulus, whether physical (heat, cold, humidity, a stuffy, steamy atmosphere or pungent smells) or psychological (fear, an insult, a compliment, or even the sigh after relief of tension). Many patients experience symptoms on relaxing before the television or on holiday. It has been shown [16] that approximately one third of normal people react excessively to a respiratory stimulus, and it is probably from these hyperreactors that sufferers are recruited. The result of such an excessive response is invariably a fluctuation and fall in arterial P_{CO_2} (fig. 2, 3) which, acting upon the brain and nervous system, can produce profound changes in bodily and mental function. Thirdly, there is great variation between individuals, both as to the degree of hypocarbia produced by overbreathing, and in the individual response to that hypocarbia.

Herein lies the possibility of confusion and overlap between hyperventilation and allergic reactions. The hyperventilation response readily becomes a conditioned reflex to any stimulus *perceived* as noxious; the 'allergic' reaction may be provoked either by non-perceived stimuli (e.g. a high pollen count) or by perceived danger (e.g. the asthmatic who develops spasm on finding himself without his inhaler or in a room in which he *thinks* there is a cat).

Figure 4 is instructive. The patient was a young woman with definite asthma. The asthma had started following an episode when she had found herself trapped in a small room with a large and savage dog. Following this, she developed both asthma and dog phobia. The respiration was monitored with an impedance spirometer, using electrodes applied to the thorax. The tracing shows the breathing during recall under hypnosis of the original traumatic incident. Bronchospasm developed and the experiment was terminated.

Physiological Changes Produced by Hyperventilation

Overbreathing 'blows off' excessive quantities of carbon dioxide and so lowers the arterial carbon dioxide tension (Pa_{CO_2}), i.e. it produces hypocarbia. When sustained, a respiratory alkalosis results, since carbon

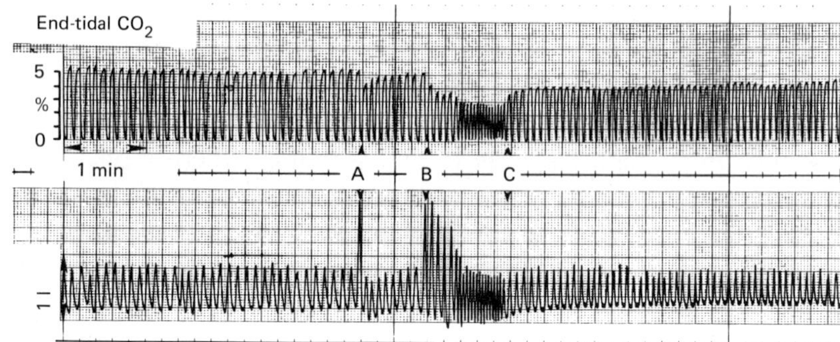

Fig. 2. Normal breathing (lower trace), with simultaneous breath by breath record of CO_2 concentration in expired air sampled at the mouth, to show the effect of a single deep breath or sigh (A) and repeated sighs and rapid breathing (B). Note: (1) regular tidal excursions during spontaneous breathing; (2) considerable fall in end-tidal CO_2 produced by single deep breath; (3) rapid fall in end-tidal CO_2 produced by 6 deep breaths, and prolonged recovery time. The end-tidal air, being in equilibrium with alveolar air, reflects instantaneous values of CO_2 in the pulmonary venous and arterial blood.

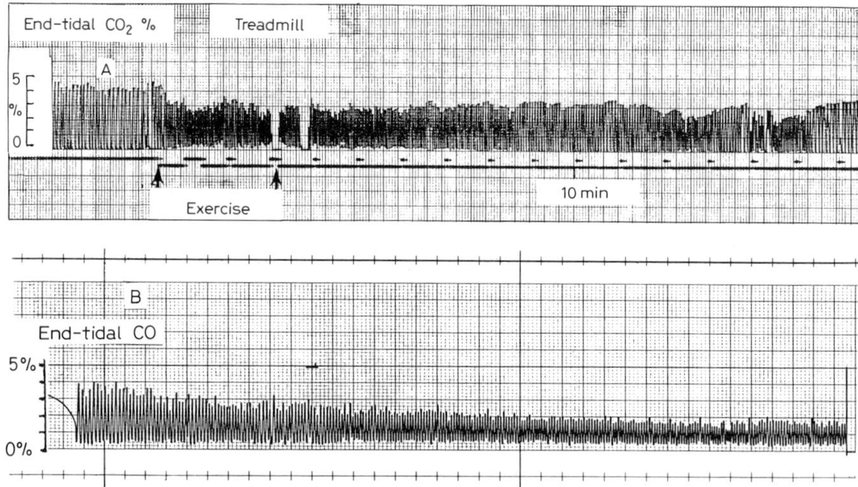

Fig. 3. A End-tidal tracing from patient with 'cardiac neurosis' when faced with treadmill exercise test. Note: Hyperventilation commences *before* exercise starts, with profound fall in end-tidal P_{CO_2}. Patient could not continue for more than 3 min. Recovery took 20 min. Heart and lungs were normal. *B* Agoraphobic. Note: (1) the initial low value of end-tidal CO_2 (about half normal), and the continued fall during the 10-min test; (2) the rapid respirations, and final rate of 32 breaths/min.

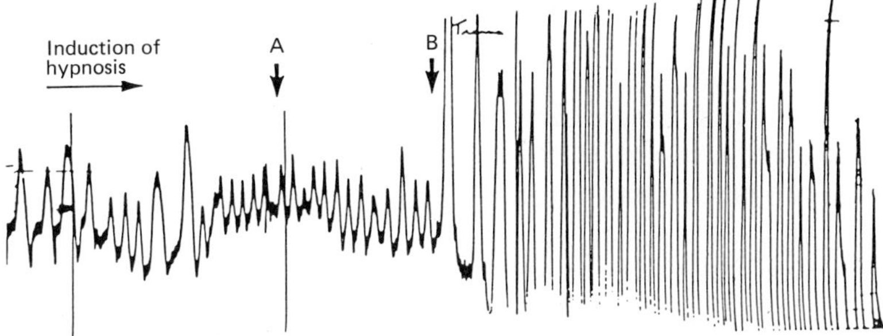

Fig. 4. This tracing (see text) was taken from a young woman who developed asthma whenever in the presence of a dog. The response here is clearly phobic. The tracing was taken many years ago and it is not known whether she was truly allergic. Following induction of a trance, she was reminded of the original incident (A). At B she was asked to relive the experience.

dioxide is acidic. It has therefore been assumed that one should find evidence of a respiratory alkalosis or low arterial carbon dioxide in sufferers from chronic habitual hyperventilation. This is not necessarily so. Unequivocally low levels of carbon dioxide were found in little more than half the cases personally observed and one third were within normal limits, the remainder being equivocal [12]. This inconstancy of relation between symptoms and respiratory alkalosis has led many influential observers [15] to discount its role in one of the commonest manifestations of chronic hyperventilation – Da Costa's syndrome. *Wood's* [15] view seems to have prevailed in England so that few except the rare and florid forms of hyperventilation are recognized here.

Advances in neurophysiological knowledge, however, have shown that it is not alkalosis (i.e. a raised pH) which is the key factor; it is the fluctuation in concentration of the carbon dioxide molecule itself (fluctuating hypocarbia), acting directly on nervous tissue, which causes symptoms [17]. The symptom complexes under discussion cover an enormously wide variety of somatic disturbance and organ dysfunction – particularly cardiac and gastro-intestinal, often suggesting some organic disease. Hyperventilation can justly be said to have displaced syphilis as 'the great mimic'. It also embraces a spectrum of psychological disorders including anxiety, depression, disturbed mentation, phobias, 'unreal' states, depersonalisation and even hallucinations. Most of the components of an acute schizoidal reaction can be produced by hyperventilation [18].

The common pathway to this plethora of symptoms is the nervous system; it is therefore necessary to review those aspects of neurophysiology where the action of carbon dioxide is most relevant. The necessarily brief review given here is drawn from *Wyke* [19] and from personal communication with the author of that work.

It is widely (but erroneously) believed that neuronal function is modulated by the pH of the cerebro-spinal fluid. It is not. The hydrogen ion is bound to a water molecule, and the total diameter of this hydrated proton is greater than that of neuronal pores; thus it can only traverse neuronal membranes extremely slowly. A change of pH in the extracellular fluid does not influence the pH value within the neurone if the P_{CO_2} is held constant. Carbon dioxide, on the other hand, passes freely through neuronal pores; it diffuses faster even than water. A fall of ambient P_{CO_2} is immediately followed by a migration of CO_2 from the neurone, with a consequent rise in intraneuronal pH, resulting in an increase in neuronal activity, and increased discharge through associated nerve fibres. Changes also occur in ionized calcium and in the transport of sodium and potassium ions; these, however, are secondary to, and contingent upon, the change in P_{CO_2}. A very slight fall in P_{CO_2} of a few millimetres of mercury can produce a measurable effect. It must be emphasized that the *only* external factor which can directly affect the intraneuronal pH is a change in the P_{CO_2} of the extracellular fluid. More profound decreases in Pa_{CO_2} cause changes in intracellular metabolism which later depress activity so that at very low Pa_{CO_2} levels, the neurone becomes inert. However, the initial effect on the motor projection systems from the cortex is excitation, with increased tone in the somatic musculature and increased stretch reflexes, expressed clinically as tension. Similarly there is increased sensory excitability: sounds seem louder, lights brighter.

There is a specific effect on facilitatory synapses involved in somatic motor reflex arcs, e.g. pupil and tendon reflexes: synaptic transmission is speeded up, thereby shortening reflex reaction times.

A complex effect on the automatic nervous system results in a picture of sympathetic dominance: dilated pupils, cold extremities, palmar and axillary sweating and tachycardia. Sympathetic-parasympathetic imbalance probably accounts for the variety of visceral disturbance encountered: bloating, belching, abdominal discomfort and dysmenorrhoea, to name but a few. There is, as in all aspects of this complex picture, considerable variation between one person and another as to which dysfunction is most troublesome at a given time.

Thus, moderate degrees of overbreathing, as in the classical ‘fight or flight’ situation, produce increased motor excitability, quickened reflexes and heightened sensory perception of light (night vision improves) and of sound (photophobia and hyperacusis are not uncommon, though seldom complained of spontaneously). The primitive survival value is obvious. However, when hypocarbia becomes very severe, as in the gross overbreathing of a panic attack, many of these responses become extinguished – in extreme cases progressing to stupor. Hence the phenomenon of paralysis by fright.

Cerebral hypoxia is a most important element in this response. Carbon dioxide is the chief controller of cerebral blood flow [20]. Hypocarbia diminishes cerebral blood flow by vasoconstriction and thus diminishes all higher cerebral activity. Inhibitions are diminished; the patient may be overemotional, or suffer outbreaks of violent behaviour; concentration, memory and cerebration are impaired (‘my head feels full of cotton wool’); depersonalisation or a feeling of unreality and delusions (usually mild), are common; hallucinations may occur but must be cautiously enquired for, since there is a frequent unspoken fear of insanity. The hypoxia is compounded by the shift to the left of the dissociation curve of haemoglobin for oxygen: the Bohr effect [21]. The lesser effects of cerebral hypoxia are probably the commonest: dizziness, faintness, and various disturbances of vision. Such effects can usually be reproduced in susceptible individuals, within 1 min of voluntary hyperventilation.

In young normal adults, the critical threshold for the onset of cerebral vasoconstriction is as little as 2 mm Hg. The fall in cerebral blood flow is not linear, however, for, as the brain becomes more hypoxic, there is an increased production of potassium ion and lactic acid, which are potent vasodilators. Hence, with deepening hypocarbia, the vasoconstrictive effect is offset by these vasodilators. One must stress the extreme variability between individuals with regard to this vascular response. A small proportion of individuals are remarkably insensitive in this respect, and it is in these that diagnosis by the provocation test may be the most difficult.

There are, however, more direct links between hyperventilation and true allergy. Hyperventilation has been shown to cause an increased output of histamine [22]. Since hypocarbia lowers the concentration of calcium ions and modulates the transmembranal flux of sodium and potassium ions [23], it would appear likely that this is due to destabilisation of mast cells. Clinically, among the population of hyperventilators personally observed, the incidence of 'allergic' phenomena appeared much higher than in normal breathers.

Headaches, spanning the whole spectrum from simple headache to classical migraine, feature prominently in the symptomatology of hyperventilation. The classical migraine aura is a set of typical hyperventilation symptoms. It is known to be associated with cerebral vasoconstriction, and hypocarbia is the principal agent known to produce the latter. Moreover, the changes in blood flow produced by hyperventilation in the intracranial parts of the carotid system are opposite to those produced in the extracranial part [19, pp. 122–124]; indeed, the reduction in cerebral flow is accompanied by a general increase in skeletal muscle flow. There is clearly overlap between the common headache of hyperventilators, the histamine headache, that produced by food to which the patient is allergic, and that produced when the patient (often in a restaurant – a situation which tends to provoke hyperventilation) thinks he has eaten something to which he may be allergic.

Diagnosis and Treatment

The key to diagnosis is awareness of the very high incidence and the protean symptomatology of hyperventilation. Older surveys suggested that hyperventilators constituted 10% of patients seeking medical advice. It is probable that this is a considerable underestimate. 'Neurotic' illness (while difficult to quantify) has, in various surveys, been shown to account for about one third of medical consultations [24]. Since the symptomatology is the same, it seems likely that hyperventilation is either the prime cause, or is playing a major part in maintaining symptoms. It should be among the first (instead of the last) diagnoses to be considered where the history does not clearly indicate an organic disease. Since many symptoms are not volunteered by the patient, direct enquiry should be made for common (but often mild) symptoms like dizziness, faintness or unsteadiness, blurred or distorted vision, paraesthesiae, air hunger, gasping or excessive sighing, belching or difficulty in swallowing, and tension pains, which the patient often rationalizes away. Psychic disturbances (anxiety or depression, tension, depersonalisation, phobias and panic attacks) are often not mentioned because of the unspoken dread of insanity. There is often an irrational fear of sudden death.

The presence of hyperventilation should not, however, be taken to exclude organic disease, since the two may co-exist. Prudent measures to exclude the latter should always be taken. However, the shunting of patients from one specialist department to another, in the hope of turning up some physical abnormality, is to be deplored. The involvement of multiple systems is a highly suggestive clue, as are frequent deep sighs during consultation, with moistening of the lips and harsh unproductive cough. Prolonged auscultation of the chest, with rapid deep breaths, will often start symptoms off. Often the patient will recognize a self-portrait when confronted with table I. The rapid, upper thoracic, breathing with frequent sighs (often heard as the physician turns from the patient to the notes) is usually obvious at a glance to the physician attuned to the diagnosis.

The most immediate diagnostic test is the reproduction of symptoms which the patient recognizes as similar to those which occur spontaneously, by forced deep breathing from 1 to 3 min at a rate of 30–40 breaths/min (normals will also get symptoms, but do not recognize them as symptoms which occur spontaneously). This test, properly performed, will be positive in about 80% of patients. It is most likely to be equivocal in those who do not readily develop symptoms of cerebral vasoconstriction. Spot checks of Pa_{CO_2} are diagnostic in only half the patients and in the author's opinion not worth doing unless to persuade the patient. A spirogram showing characteristic irregularities is helpful, but the trained eye can detect these on inspection.

Treatment by teaching a slow, regular, diaphragmatic breathing, with suppression of upper thoracic movement and of sighing respirations, results in complete abolition of symptoms in nearly 80% of cases, and marked improvement in a further 15%. The patient needs also to be taught relaxation, and how to deal with those aspects of his personality which expose him to excessive stress. Most women have markedly perfectionist tendencies, and the type A male [24] predominates.

In acute, severe attacks, resort may be had to the time-honoured rebreathing from a paper bag. Usually, however, calm instruction to quieten the breathing will restore the patient. Many, however, are comforted by carrying an appropriate bag for use in an emergency.

Space precludes detailed discussion of the treatment regime used in the author's series, for which the reader is referred to articles by *Lum* [26] and *Cluff* [27]. A basically similar approach is described by *Innocenti* [28].

Concluding Remarks

The symptomatology of hyperventilation is protean and may involve any organ or body system. Similar symptom complexes are often found in patients who appear to be having allergic reactions. From experience of over 2,300 cases, the clinical features and breathing characteristics found in hyperventilation syndromes have been reviewed. Physiological tests have been used to exclude lung disease and to document the aberrant breathing patterns and the excessive lability of the lowered arterial carbon dioxide. An attempt has been made to show how hyperventilation can become a conditioned reflex response when the patient experiences a situation which is considered to be noxious or harmful.

The hyperventilation reaction is disproportionately large in about one third of the population, and in these cases the likelihood of experiencing hypocarbic symptoms in certain situations is enhanced. When such a reaction does occur, there is a strong temptation to attribute it to something in that situation. For example, a patient who experiences faintness, dizziness, nausea or migraine in a warm, crowded and stuffy restaurant or at a dinner party (conditions conducive to hyperventilation) may become phobic about such situations or, equally, may consider that an allergy to food is involved. Repetition of the reaction in similar circumstances is likely to set up a conditioned reflex response and to reinforce an original mis-diagnosis of food allergy. Such patients are to be regarded as suffering from pseudo-food allergy [c.f. *Pearson and Rix,* this volume]. The breathing pattern of hyperventilating patients is quite characteristic but seldom recognized by clinicians. The fluctuating hypocarbia produced by this type of breathing acts upon the central nervous system to produce the symptoms as described.

References

1 Darwin, C.: Expression of emotions in man and animals (Murray, London 1872).
2 Cannon, W.B.: The mechanism of emotional disturbance of bodily functions. New Engl. J. Med. *198:* 877 (1928).
3 Christie, R.V.: Some types of respiration in the neuroses. Q. Jl Med. *16:* 427 (1935).
4 Laurens, A. du: A discourse of the preservation of the sight; of melancholoke diseases; of rheumes and of old age (London 1595).
5 Haldane, J.S.; Poulton, E.P.: The effects of want of oxygen on respiration. Proc. physiol. Soc. *37:* 390 (1908).

6 White, P.D.; Hahn, R.G.: The symptom of sighing in cardiovascular diagnosis. Am. J. med. Sci. *177:* 179 (1929).
7 Kerr, W.J.; Dalton, J.W.; Gliebe, P.A.: Some physical phenomena associated with the anxiety states and their relation to hyperventilation. Ann. intern. Med. *11:* 96 (1937).
8 Engel, G.L.; Ferris, E.B.; Logan, M.; Hyperventilation: analysis of clinical symptomatology. Ann. intern. Med. *27:* 683 (1947).
9 Rice, R.L.: Symptom patterns of the hyperventilation syndrome. Am. J. Med. *8:* 691 (1950).
10 Lewis, B.I.: Mechanism and management of hyperventilation syndromes. Biochem. Clin. *4:* 89 (1964).
11 Tucker, W.I.: Hyperventilation in differential diagnosis. Med. Clins N. Am. *47:* 491 (1963).
12 Lum, L.C.: The syndrome of chronic habitual hyperventilation. in Hill, Modern trends in psychosomatic medicine; 3rd ed., pp. 196–230 (Butterworths, London 1976).
13 Magarian, G.J.: Hyperventilation syndromes: infrequently recognized common expressions of anxiety and stress. Medicine, Baltimore *61:* 219 (1982).
14 Gottlieb, B.: Non-organic disease in medical out-patients. Update *1:* 917 (1969).
15 Wood, P.: Da Costa's syndrome (or effort syndrome). The mechanism of the somatic manifestations. Br. med. J., 24 May, 805 (1941).
16 Lambertsen, C.J.: Carbon dioxide and respiration in acid-base homoeostasis. Anesthesiology *21:* 642 (1960).
17 Lum, L.C.: Hyperventilation and anxiety state. J. R. Soc. Med. *74:* 1 (1981).
18 Allen, T.E.; Agus, B.: Hyperventilation leading to hallucinations. Am. J. Psychol. *125:* 632 (1968).
19 Wyke, B.: Brain function and metabolic disorders (Butterworths, London 1963).
20 Lennox, W.G.; Gibbs, F.A.; Gibbs, E.L.: The relationship in man of cerebral activity to blood flow and to blood constituents. J. Neurol. Psychiat. Lond. *1:* 211 (1938).
21 Bohr, C.; Hasselbach, K.A.; Krogh, A.: Über einen in biologischer Beziehung wichtigen Einfluss, den die Kohlensäurespannung des Blutes auf dessen Sauerstoffbindung übt. Skand. Archiv. Physiol. *16*, p. 402 (1904).
22 Kontos, H.A.; Richardson, D.W.; Raper, A.J.; Zubair-ul-Hassan; Patterson, J.L., Jr.: Mechanisms of action of hypocapnic alkalosis on limb blood vessels in man and dog. Am. J. Physiol. *223:* 1296 (1972).
23 Wyke, B.: Principles of general neurology (Elsevier, Amsterdam 1969).
24 Eysenck, H.J.: You and neurosis (Scientific Book Club, London 1977).
25 Friedman, M.; Rosenman, R.: Association of specific overt behaviour pattern with blood and cardiovascular findings. J. Am. med. Ass. *169:* 1286 (1959).
26 Lum, L.C.: Physiological principles in the treatment of hyperventilation syndromes. Tijdschr. geneesmiddelenonderzoek (J. Drug Res.) *8:* 1867–1872 (1983).
27 Cluff, R.A.: Chronic hyperventilation and its treatment by physiotherapy. J. R. Soc. Med. (in press 1984).
28 Innocenti, D.M.: Chronic hyperventilation syndrome; in Downie, Cash's textbook of chest, heart and vascular disorders for physiotherapists; 3rd ed., pp. 356–365 (Faber & Faber, London 1983).

L.C. Lum, MA, MB, FRCP, FRACP, Papworth and Addenbrooke's Hospitals, Cambridge, CB3 8BX (England)

PAR. Pseudo-Allergic Reactions. Involvement of Drugs and Chemicals, vol. 4, pp. 120–137 (Karger, Basel 1985)

Malignant Hyperpyrexia

P. Jane Halsall, F. Richard Ellis

University Department of Anaesthesia, St. James's Hospital, Leeds, UK

In 1960 a young Australian man presented with a fractured leg. He was less concerned about the necessary surgery than about the anaesthetic, as 11 relatives had died as a result of ether anaesthesia. Subsequently he survived a reaction which came to be known as malignant hyperpyrexia (MH, or malignant hyperthermia) [13]. Since then, the condition has become widely recognised and is now a major cause of death in otherwise fit, healthy young adults. Although it occurs more frequently in young males, this is a reflection of the differing life-styles rather than a true sex difference.

The development of an MH reaction in response to anaesthesia is characterised by an unexplained tachycardia or arrhythmia associated with tachypnoea, in addition to a rapid increase in core temperature of the order of 5–6 °C/h. Frequently muscle rigidity also occurs. Biochemical signs of MH include a metabolic acidosis, hyperkalaemia and increased CO_2 production. These signs represent a marked stimulation of the metabolic processes in the order of 5–6 times basal levels.

Incidence

The incidence of MH has been variably quoted from 1:20,000–1:200,000. However, with better recognition of the disease, it is now thought to be about 1:50,000. The mortality rate has decreased from 70% to less than 50% but is still depressingly high, this despite claims that, with the introduction of a suitable intravenous preparation of dantrolene sodium, a hydantoin compound, the problems of MH had been resolved.

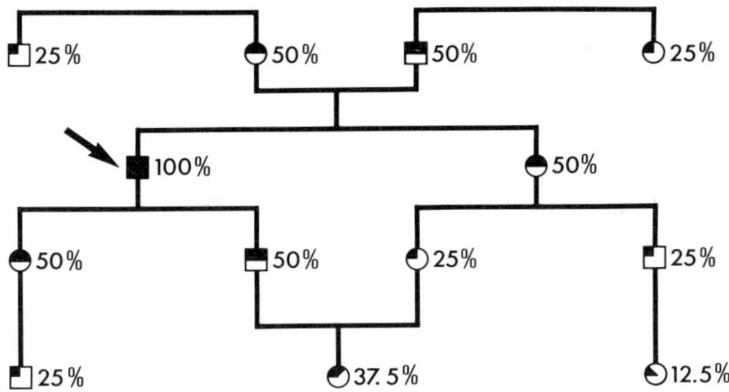

Fig. 1. The theoretical probability (percentage) of inheriting MH before family screening studies have been initiated. The proband is indicated by the arrow.

Inheritance

The evidence suggests that the susceptibility to MH is inherited as an autosomal-dominant trait. A theoretical pedigree showing the chance of inheriting the MH predisposition is shown in figure 1. MH was originally described as a disease with variable expression, firstly because some patients failed to develop MH on exposure to the triggering agents and secondly due to creatinine phosphokinase (CPK) prediction which proved to be unreliable. Failure to react to the triggering agents is now thought to be due to other factors, particularly 'stress' (see later).

Ideally, all patients, excepting referred probands attending for MH screening, should be restricted to those having a 50% probability of MH, unless there are good reasons why a key relative has to be omitted. Using this criterion, roughly 50% of all patients can be shown to be susceptible to MH (MHS), thus bearing out the theory of autosomal-dominant inheritance.

'Triggering' Agents

Many drugs have been implicated as 'trigger' agents in MH. The most important ones are the depolarising muscle relaxants, e.g. suxamethonium, and the volatile anaesthetic gases, e.g. halothane. Furthermore, it has long been known that some drugs with adrenergic properties used in psychiatry as antidepressants can produce fever, probably through a central pathway involving the hypothalamus.

In addition, neuroleptic malignant syndrome, first described by *Delay and Deniker* [10] in 1968, is associated with a variety of antipsychotic agents, particularly the neuroleptics and possibly the phenothiazines. The aetiology is unknown, but it has been linked with lethal catatonia and may occur following the combined use of lithium and the neuroleptics. Features of the disease include severe dyskinesia, temperature elevation, tachycardia, blood pressure fluctuation and dyspnoea. Recently *Coons* et al. [9] have described a case of neuroleptic malignant syndrome which was improved by the use of dantrolene.

The role of lignocaine as a trigger drug for MH is controversial. Although frequently reported as a triggering agent [3], lignocaine epidural injections have been used to prevent an MH reaction in susceptible swine [33]. It has been suggested that amide-linked local anaesthetics should be avoided in MHs patients [3], but in our experience one example of this type of local anaesthetic agent, bupivacaine, has been quite uneventful.

Muscle Rigidity

A common, and often first, presenting sign of MH is muscle spasm following suxamethonium. This may be localised to the masseter muscles, but can be more generalised. Indeed, 1 MH patient died due to hypoxia following gross muscle rigidity after suxamethonium which prevented adequate ventilation [personal observation]. Frequently, a minor abnormal reaction to suxamethonium is thought to be due to extravascular injection, insufficient dosage or hydrolysis of the drug, and a further dose is administered which usually precipitates a more definite reaction. Conversely, when the anaesthetic is abandoned at this juncture, what is the probability of it being a true MH reaction? In a survey of 277 probands screened by this Unit, 100 developed suxamethonium-induced spasm. Two thirds of these were shown to have MH and of these 11% had no other signs of MH, 14% had minimal signs and 75% had definite signs. Of the one third of probands not susceptible to MH but who developed suxamethonium-induced spasm, 25% were shown to have another disorder (e.g. myotonia) and in 33% no other explanation of the problem was found. A

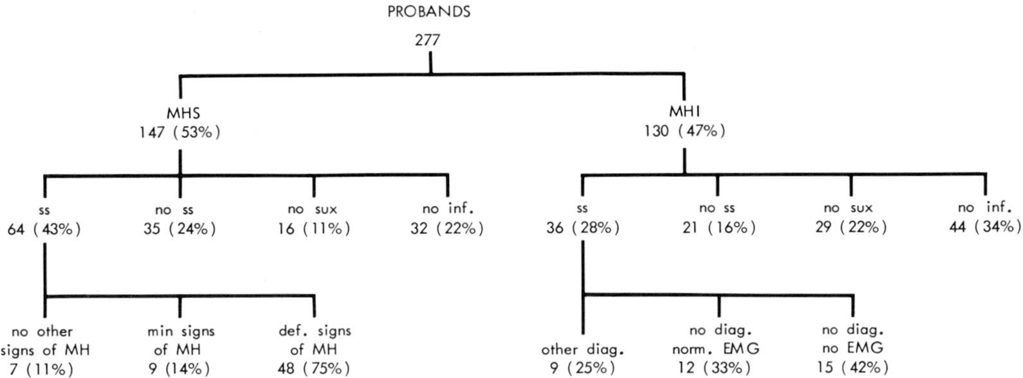

Fig. 2. Incidence of suxamethonium-induced muscle spasm (SS) in MH referrals. See text for details. MHS = Susceptible to MH; MHI = insusceptible to MH; SUX = suxamethonium.

further group of patients (42%) had an incomplete investigation as an electromyogram (EMG) had been omitted. A summary of these findings is shown in figure 2 [16].

Anthropometric Features

Denborough et al. [11] originally described the Evans myopathy after a family exhibiting several myopathic features and many other workers have commented on the muscular build of these patients. In particular, there is frequently marked enlargement of the muscles in the lateral part of the thigh (fig. 3) and in addition they are more heavily muscled [7]. Despite these muscle abnormalities, which are frequently seen as gross histological changes (see later), these patients are very active and often excel at sports. There is a greater incidence of other musculo-skeletal problems in patients with MH. 50 consecutive probands, for example, were having surgery for the conditions listed in table I when the MH reaction occurred.

From this, it can be seen that musculo-skeletal abnormalities are comparatively prominent. From the incidence statistics, a Bayesean analysis can provide a priori probability of MH occurring, and this would include the following factors: musculo-skeletal abnormalities (e.g. squint, hernia, cartilage problems, kyphoscoliosis), anthropometric observations,

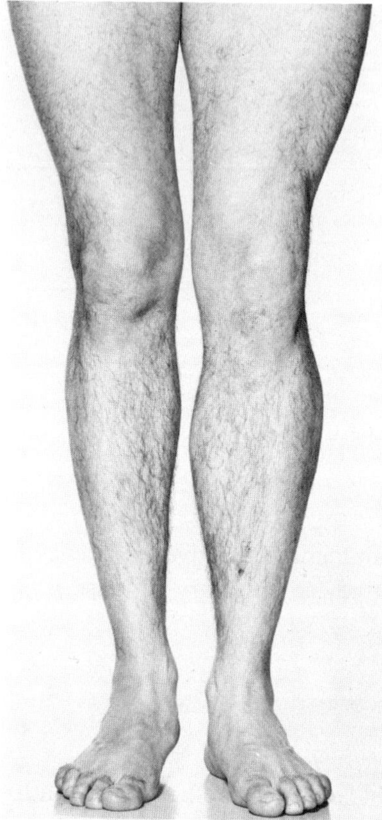

Fig. 3. Enlargement of the lateral compartment of the thighs in MHS patients.

abnormal anaesthetic family history, and biochemical abnormalities (e.g. high CPK). Using a simplified analysis, *Wilson and Ellis* [42] reported that, as 15% of MH probands have squints and as 1.5% of the general population have squints, the likelihood of a squint patient developing MH is increased by 15:1.5, that is, 10 times.

Treatment of a Reaction

Diagnosis commences with adequate monitoring of all patients subjected to anaesthesia. Only in this way can trends in the patient's condi-

Table I. Operation being performed at the time of the MH reaction

	Number	%
Trauma	10	20
Squint and ptosis	9	18
Cartilage	5	10
Appendix	5	10
Kyphoscoliosis	4	8
Tonsils and adenoids	4	8
Hernia	3	6
Dental	3	6
Abdominal	1	2
Others	6	12

tion be easily followed. Temperature monitoring is essential, although a rise in temperature may be a late sign. Often the first sign of things going wrong, in the absence of suxamethonium-induced spasm, is an inappropriate tachycardia and tachypnoea. When CO_2 levels are also being monitored, these may also be raised. Once the diagnosis of MH has been made, treatment needs to be active and swift.

All triggering drugs should be withdrawn, including anaesthetic equipment contaminated with anaesthetic vapours. Blood samples should be taken for the measurement of blood gases, K^+ and CPK. Intravenous dantrolene should be given in an initial dose of 1 mg/kg and, in addition, large doses of steroids (e.g. solumedrone 1 g). Blood gases and serum K^+ should be corrected as required and, although K^+ levels may be very high at the commencement of the reaction, in the later stages these can fall considerably as large amounts of K^+ are lost in the urine. Massive breakdown of the muscle tissue, as well as producing excess K^+, also produces myoglobin. This can block the renal tubules causing renal failure due to acute tubular necrosis. Mannitol may be used to promote diuresis and the first voided sample should be analysed for myoglobin. Renal failure is reversible with the use of dialysis but may take many weeks.

Only if MH is treated early can the patient have any chance of survival. Claims that MH as a life-threatening condition had been resolved following the introduction of a suitable intravenous preparation of dantrolene have been shown to be incorrect. Dantrolene cannot reverse MH once it has progressed too far. When the patient has fully recovered, he should be referred for investigation by muscle biopsy to prove the diagnosis. This

Table II. Differential diagnosis of MH

Pyrexia	*Suxamethonium spasm*
Endogenous toxins	Real
Blood transfusion	Myotonic muscle disease
Head injury, brain tumour or cerebrovascular accident	Denervation
Atropine overdose	Apparent
Convulsions	Failure to relax
Thyroid crisis	Extravascular injection
Peripheral circulatory failure	Inactive suxamethonium
Some drugs used in psychiatry	Light anaesthesia
	Fibrosis
	Myoglobinuria
	Haematonia
	Muscle spasm
	Familial paroxysmal rhabdomyolysis
	McArdle's disease or the glycogenoses

is necessary because of the implications of the diagnosis to the patient and the family. The possible differential diagnoses for MH, including (a) pyrexia, (b) muscle spasm resulting from suxamethonium and (c) myoglobinuria are shown in table II.

Family Investigations

In vitro screening for MH developed following the demonstration that skeletal muscle from suspected cases of MH produced abnormal contractures when exposed to caffeine [31, 32]. Caffeine causes contracture in normal muscle but only at high concentrations, and thus evidence for MH depends upon demonstrating a greater sensitivity to caffeine. Subsequently, *Ellis* et al. [19] showed that MHS muscle developed contractures when exposed to halothane in the tissue bath at 37 °C whereas normal muscle did not. Previous workers had not shown this because the muscle had been kept at room temperature rather than at physiological temperature. Despite screening patients for MH by in vitro tests for nearly 15 years, there is still much heated debate over the interpretation of the tests and also of the exact protocol used. This results in many difficulties in understanding the significance of research data. Recently, a European MH

Group was founded with the initial aim both of standardising the testing protocol and its interpretation (thus providing a consensus for the criteria needed to diagnose MH) and of allowing for the collaboration of data [20].

At present, Leeds is the only centre in the UK offering screening facilities to patients, although there are several centres interested in porcine MH. Patients are admitted to hospital for 2 nights. Pre-operatively, an electrocardiogram (ECG), chest X-ray, haemoglobin and electrolytes are investigated and photography of their muscle build made. The biopsy, from the left vastus internus muscle, is performed under a specially developed modified general anaesthesia. This includes intermittent thiopentone and fentanyl with 50% nitrous oxide in oxygen, without any premedication.

Selection of Patients

When a patient dies, the nearest, most appropriate relative is tested. When the patient is a child less than age 10 years, the parents are investigated because of dubious in vitro results in young children. When the first parent is shown to be MHS, the second parent is assumed to be normal, due to the rarity of the condition. When the first parent is negative, the second parent is biopsied. Using figure 1, the chances of other family members being affected can be predicted and those members having a 50% probability are offered muscle biopsy screening. In this way, all affected members of a family can be identified. Although this may seem a rather laborious and costly procedure, the alternative is more horrific as a typical theoretical family may contain 628 people. This is an enormous number to label as MHS when only 8% of the family need to be investigated by muscle biopsy to identify the 3.8% who will be affected (fig. 4). In the past, high resting CPK values were thought to indicate susceptibility to MH [29] and this idea was greeted enthusiastically as a convenient screening test. However, CPK values have now been shown to be inadequate for screening as there are many false positives and more seriously, false negatives [14].

In vitro Tests

Muscle samples are taken across the motor point (a painful procedure) and are about 3 cm long and 2–3 mm thick. Four specimens are given to

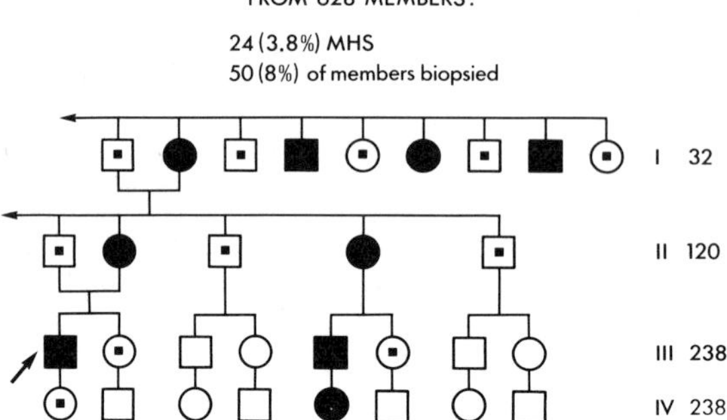

Fig. 4. A theoretical family tree indicating the number of individuals needed to be investigated to identify those with MH susceptibility.

the pathologist for electron microscopy, block De-Castro, De-Castro and cryostat and four specimens are retained for the in vitro tests. These are placed in fresh Krebs solution, transported to the laboratory, aerated with 95% oxygen and 5% carbon dioxide (carbogen) and stored at room temperature while the tests are being carried out. A sample is placed in the tissue bath and one end attached to a strain gauge. The tissue bath, maintained at 37 °C, is continuously perfused with aerated Krebs solution. The strain gauge is mounted on a micrometer stage which can be moved vertically by a constant speed motor. The muscle is electrically stimulated supramaximally to ensure viability. A schematic diagram of the apparatus is shown in figure 5. Three specimens of muscle are exposed to different concentrations of halothane and caffeine using a set protocol [20]. A comparison of a negative and positive dynamic halothane result is shown in fig. 6 for samples from 2 patients [18].

Histology

There are several, non-specific histological abnormalities associated with MH [28]. Not all patients with in vitro evidence of MH have histological abnormalities. This finding led to the suggestion that the inheritance of MH was multifactorial [14], although this is now disputed. The abnormalities found in MHS muscle include internal nuclei (fig. 7), 'moth-

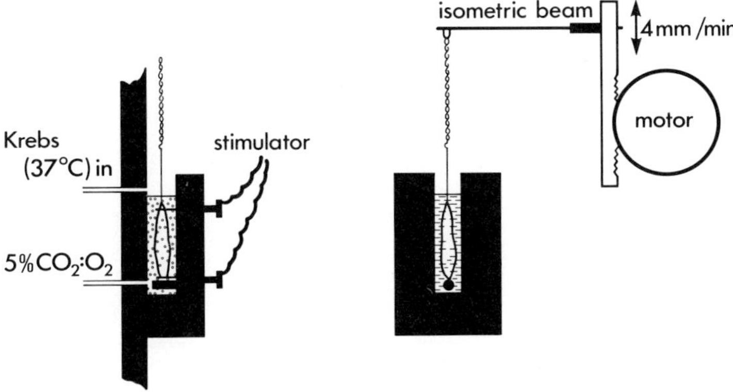

Fig. 5. Schematic diagram of the tissue bath in coronal and sagittal sections used for screening for MH susceptibility.

eaten' fibres, cores (fig. 8), fibre hypertrophy, fibre splitting and a variation in fibre size.

Having established the diagnosis using these tests, the patient (or relative) is given both a booklet describing the condition and a warning card of the drugs which should be avoided, and encouraged to join the Medic-Alert Foundation.

Anaesthesia for MHS Patients

MHS patients can receive safe anaesthesia for necessary surgery, providing certain guidelines are followed [5]. These include a good working knowledge of MH by the anaesthetist, adequate temperature and ECG monitoring, cooling facilities, avoidance of the triggering drugs, and appropriate drug treatment on hand. We do not advocate the use of prophylactic dantrolene as do some workers, as it is unpleasant for the patient and not without side-effects. During anaesthesia for muscle biopsy, dantrolene cannot be given as it interferes with the results of the in vitro tests.

The avoidance of the triggering drugs, particularly suxamethonium, sometimes makes anaesthesia difficult and hazardous in certain situations. This is why many anaesthetists postpone operative procedures until MH can be confirmed by muscle biopsy.

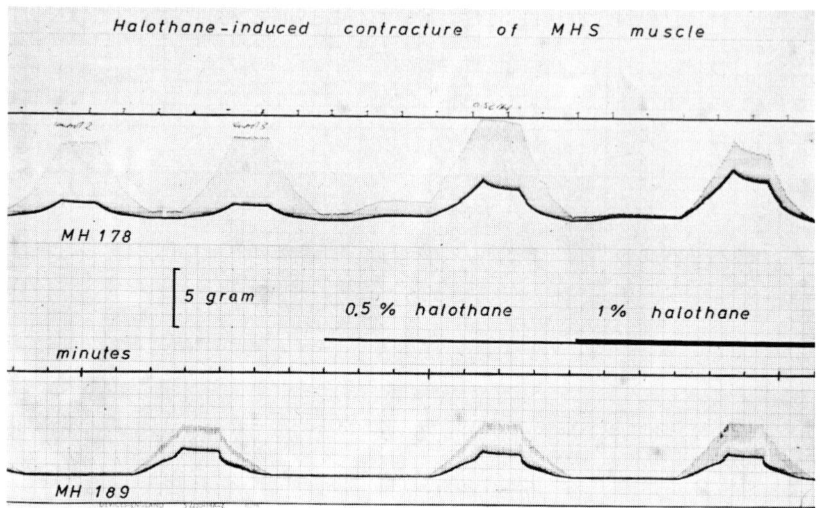

Fig. 6. The in vitro dynamic halothane test. A comparison of a positive (upper trace) and normal (lower trace) in vitro result to the dynamic halothane test. The first peak is the control curve, which is compared with the curve obtained with different concentrations of halothane. A normal result is indicated by a decrease in the curve as the muscle relaxes with halothane. An increase in the curve caused by the muscle contracting in response to halothane indicates a positive result.

The drugs which are safe to use in MH include the induction agents thiopentone and althesin. Muscle relaxation can be provided safely using pancuronium, alcuronium, and possibly atracurium. All analgesics can be used, although nitrous oxide should be restricted to 50%. Droperidol is a useful anti-emetic and the benzodiazepines are useful sedatives. Both bupivacaine and prilocaine can be used for local anaesthesia. Using combinations of these drugs, anaesthesia, local or general, can be given to MHS patients with safety.

Aetiology

MH skeletal muscle has been extensively investigated, mostly in susceptible swine and many of the results are contradictory. Ca^{++} has an important role in excitation-contraction coupling, a possible mechanism

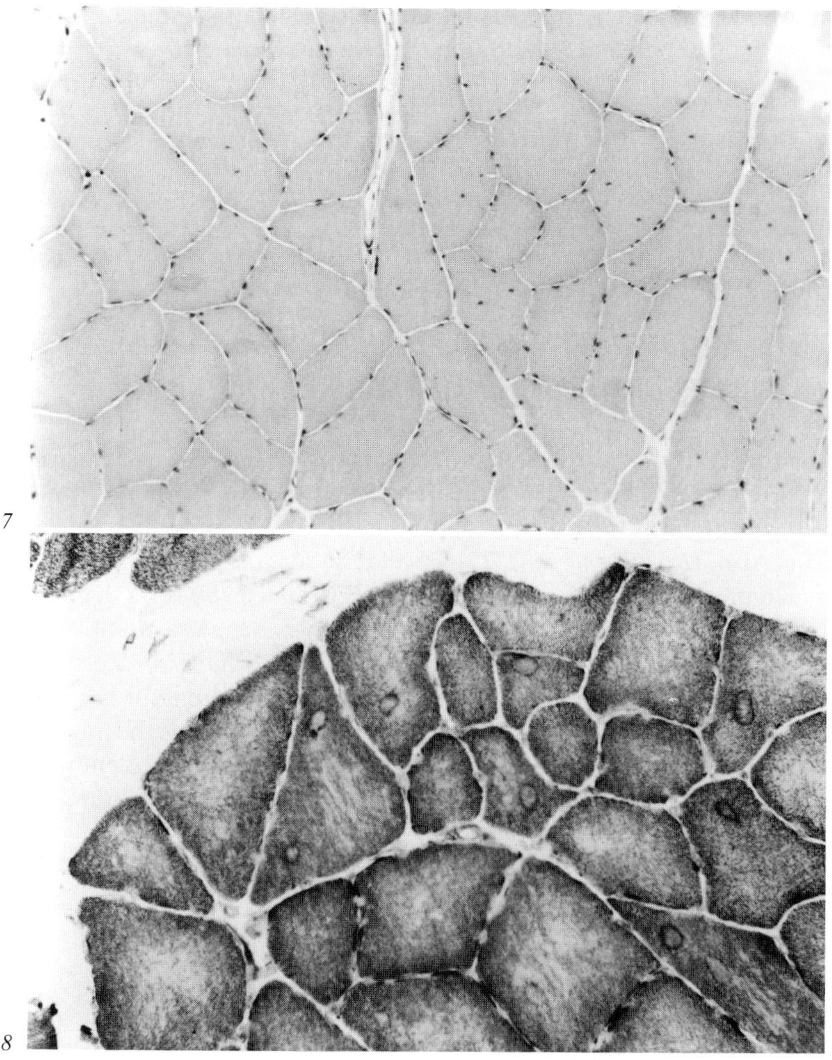

7

8

Fig. 7. Histology of the vastus internus muscle showing internal nuclei (courtesy of *Dr. D.G.F. Harriman*). × 127.

Fig. 8. Histology of the vastus internus muscle showing central cores (courtesy of *Dr. D.G.F. Harriman*). × 195.

for MH postulated by *Nelson* [40], and in cell metabolism, many enzymes being Ca^{++}-dependent. In addition, there is also a Ca^{++}-regulating protein, calmodulin. Thus the intracellular role of Ca^{++} is ubiquitous and part of the difficulties in interpreting data are the interrelationships of dynamic actions within the cell. More recently, an abnormality in the cell membrane has become accepted as the inherited defect in MH. Alterations in function of sarcolemma, 'T' tubule, sarcoplasmic reticulum or mitochondria in relation to Ca^{++} movements and actions could have marked effects on the subsequent actions within the cell.

The Sarcolemma or Plasma Membrane

Evidence that the sarcolemma is abnormal in MHS swine has been reported by *Gallant* et al. [22], who showed that halothane produced partial depolarisation of skeletal muscle which was prevented by dantrolene. Also, *Halsall and Ellis* [27] have found that dantrolene is more effective in preventing the muscle contractures produced by K^+, a depolarising ion, than those produced by caffeine and halothane in the rat. Stimulation of the membrane causes release of trigger Ca^{++}, which in turn starts the process of excitation-contraction coupling. Suxamethonium is a strongly charged drug and therefore likely to have its effects outside the muscle cell. This adds weight to the view that an abnormality at the sarcolemma exists in MH [26]. Another possibility is a defect in the Na^+/Ca^{++} pump.

The Sarcoplasmic Reticulum

By far the highest amounts of Ca^{++} are found in association with the sarcoplasmic reticulum (SR), only 10% occurring in both the sarcolemma and the mitochondria. The view that the SR is the site of the basic defect in MH was the original theory put forward by *Britt* [4], and this view is still widely held. Caffeine in low concentrations (less than 10 m*M*) produces a release of Ca^{++} from the SR stores, whereas in higher concentrations it prevents re-uptake by the SR. In addition, dantrolene inhibits caffeine contractures in muscle of the rat [27], but has a more significant effect on K^+ contractures. Further evidence has been provided by *Moulds and Denborough* [39] in humans and *Feinstein* [21] in frogs to show that procaine reverses the halothane-induced and caffeine-induced contractures in vitro. The main action of procaine probably is in preventing Ca^{++} release from the SR [2], and there has been much dispute over the role of procaine as a therapeutic agent in MH. *Nelson* at the 1982 workshop in Banff (Canada) showed that there is a lowering of threshold for Ca^{++} release by the SR in MH muscle. *Gronert* et al. [23] confirmed that changes in the SR activity occur during MH, but stated that this was not sufficient to account for the whole process. Perhaps changes in the Ca^{++} released from the sarcolemma and also changes in temperature and pH could initiate alterations in the SR, implying a secondary phenomenon.

The Mitochondria

Some authors have claimed that the respiratory properties of MHS mitochondria are different from those of normal, but others have not found this [38]. More interest has recently been taken in the role of mitochondria in the regulation of myoplasmic Ca^{++}. For example, *Cheah* [8] suggests that there is an alteration in the mitochondrial membrane permeability due to an increased amount of calmodulin, a Ca^{++}-regulating protein. This is said to be responsible for enhanced activity of phospholipase A2, resulting in excess release of Ca^{++}. The increase in myoplasmic Ca^{++} causes a further release of Ca^{++} from the SR (known as Ca^{++}-induced Ca^{++} release), thereby causing muscle rigidity and stimulation of glycolysis. Phosholipase A2 has also been shown to affect other membranes such as the sarcolemma and the SR.

Human Muscle Metabolic Studies

As part of the MH reaction involves gross disturbances in metabolism reflected by hyperpyrexia, increased CO_2 output and metabolic acidosis, metabolism of MH muscle has been studied, although great care had to be taken with the method of freezing muscle samples as it may alter the biochemical findings considerably [25]. The occurrence of rapid glycolysis during an MH response was demonstrated in swine [25] and similar findings have been shown in human MHS muscle taken during the screening biopsy. These include a significantly lower glycogen level, an increased lactate level, and a decreased ATP level [15, 17]. *Isaacs and Heffron* [30] have also reported lower ATP levels and increased glucose 6-phosphate levels. This increased rate of glycolysis has been shown to be a secondary phenomenon, being stimulated by increases in cyclic 3′,5′-adenosine monophosphate (cAMP) and active phosphorylase [17]. *Willner* et al. [41] have also reported increases in cAMP resulting from increased production due to raised adenyl cyclase activity. No change in phosphodiesterase activity, responsible for the breakdown of cAMP, was found. Furthermore, levels of adenylate kinase have not shown any major changes [37].

All these substances are intimately involved with Ca^{++} and Ca^{++}-regulating proteins. Interestingly, catecholamines (resulting from exercise and stress) and also halothane and thyroid hormones can stimulate adenyl cyclase whereas caffeine chiefly stimulates phosphodiesterase. *Mitchell and Heffron* [38] recently put forward an excellent diagrammatic summary of the metabolic changes occurring in MH.

Stress Syndrome

Certain breeds of pigs are notably susceptible to MH and develop reactions without anaesthesia, frequently dying during transportation or handling or copulation. It is a major economic problem. The role of stress as a cause of MH in humans has also been given as the reason for the variable expression of the disease. *Wingard* [43] has quoted anecdotal cases of sudden death in otherwise fit, healthy young adults, particularly in response to severe exercise. *Lister* et al. [34] observed an increase in catecholamine levels in swine during an MH reaction, a finding which was confirmed by *Gronert and Theye* [24]. Partial protection from MH was obtained by α-adrenergic blockade and conversely administration of α-agonists precipitated fatal hyperpyrexia [35]. In this way, these authors showed the importance of catecholamines in an MH reaction, the adrenal medulla making an important contribution [36]. Indirect evidence that catecholamines are involved in human MH came when *Campbell* et al. [6] showed a decrease in dietary-induced thermogenesis when MHS volunteers were exercised. This is similar to hypoxic-induced catecholamine stimulation experienced at high altitude.

This theory was expanded further when MHS volunteers were subjected to a cycling exercise stress producing a maximum heart rate of 180 beats/min. This study gave evidence of decreased vasodilation in MHS subjects and a small but important difference in core temperature. The next study involved subjecting the MHS volunteers to cold-induced stress with the use of a cooling suit similar to that used by RAF pilots. MHS patients maintained their core temperature better than did the control subjects and this was due to decreased heat loss and increased heat production [1].

Cot Deaths and MH

Denborough et al. [12] have suggested a link between cot death (sudden infant death syndrome, SIDS) and MH. In a small series of cot death families (15), one third were also found to have MH. Post-mortem examination of cot death babies has frequently shown a higher core temperature than expected and changes in the small blood vessels consistent with heat stroke have been described. Interestingly, there is a phenomenon of pen deaths in swine. Since these reports, we have questioned all our MH families regarding the incidence of cot deaths but have not found it to be greater than expected. Currently, those SIDS parents wishing to undergo tests for MH are being offered muscle biopsy. Thus the link between SIDS and MH remains unsolved at present.

Thus, malignant hyperpyrexia, elicited in humans and experimental animals by some drugs, is the consequence of a pharmacogenetic disease involving skeletal muscle and possibly 'stress' factors.

References

1 Ayling, J.S.; Currie, S.; Ellis, F.R.; Halsall, P.J.; Hay, E.E.; Hills, R.: The influence of surface cooling on body temperature and heat production in patients susceptible to malignant hyperpyrexia (Abstract). J. Physiol., Lond. (in press, 1984).

2 Bianchi, C.P.: Pharmacological actions on excitation-contraction coupling in striated muscle. Fed. Proc. *27:* 126–131 (1968).

3 Britt, B.A.: Prevention of malignant hyperthermia; in Gordon, Britt, Kalow, Malignant hyperthermia, p. 451 (Thana, Illinois 1973).

4 Britt, B.A.: Aetiology and pathophysiology of malignant hyperthermia. Fed. Proc. *38:* 44–48 (1979).

5 Cain, P.A.; Ellis, F.R.: Anaesthesia for patients susceptible to malignant hyperpyrexia. A study of pancuronium and methylprednisolone. Br. J. Anaesth. *49:* 941–944 (1977).

6 Campbell, I.T.; Ellis, F.R.; Evans, R.T.: Metabolic rate and blood hormone and metabolic levels of individuals susceptible to malignant hyperpyrexia at rest and in response to food and mild exercise. Anesthesiology *55:* 46–52 (1981).

7 Campbell, I.T.; Ellis, F.R.; Halsall, P.J.; Hogge, M.St.J.: Anthropometric studies of human subjects susceptible to malignant hyperpyrexia. Acta anaesth. scand. *26:* 363–367 (1982).

8 Cheah, K.S.: Molecular agents of malignant hyperthermia and muscular dystrophy. Biochem. Soc. Trans. (in press, 1984).

9 Coons, D.J.; Hillman, F.J.; Marshall, R.W.: Treatment of neuroleptic malignant syndrome with dantrolene sodium: a case report. Am. J. Psychiat. *139:* 944–945 (1982).

10 Delay, J.; Deniker, P.: Drug-induced extrapyramidal syndromes; in Vaiken, Burgh, Handbook of clinical neurology, vol. 6: Diseases of the basal ganglia (American Elsevier, New York 1968).

11 Denborough, M.A.; Ebeling, P.; Knig, J.O.; Zapf, P.: Myopathy and malignant hyperpyrexia. Lancet *i:* 1138–1140 (1970).

12 Denborough, M.A.; Galloway, G.J.; Hopkinson, K.C.: Malignant hyperpyrexia and sudden infant death. Lancet *ii:* 1068 (1982).

13 Denborough, M.A.; Lovell, R.R.: Anaesthetic deaths in a family. Lancet *ii:* 45 (1960).

14 Ellis, F.R.; Cain, P.A.; Harriman, D.F.G.: Multifactorial inheritance of maligant hyperpyrexia susceptibility; in Aldrete, Britt, Maligant hyperpyrexia, p. 329 (Grune & Stratton, New York 1978).

15 Ellis, F.R.; Drake, J.D.; Halsall, P.J.; Hay, E.: Increased glycolyis of muscle in unstressed patients susceptible to malignant hyperpyrexia (Abstract). Br. J. Anaesth. *54:* 1132 (1982).

16 Ellis, F.R.; Halsall, P.J.: Suxamethonium spasm: a diagnostic conundrum. Br. J. Anaesth. (in press, 1984).

17 Ellis, F.R.; Halsall, P.J.; Allam, P.; Hay, E.: A biochemical abnormality found in muscle from unstressed malignant hyperpyrexia susceptile humans. Proc. Biochem. Soc. (in press, 1984).

18 Ellis, F.R.; Harriman, D.G.F.; Currie, S.; Cain, P.A.: Screening for malignant hyperpyrexia in susceptible patients; in Aldrete, Britt, Malignant hyperthermia, p. 273 (Grune & Stratton, New York 1978).

19 Ellis, F.R.; Kearney, N.P.; Harriman, D.G.F.; Summer, D.W.; Kyei-Mensah, K.; Tyrell, J.H.; Hargreaves, J.B.; Parikh, R.K.; Mulrooney, P.L.: Screening for malignant hyperpyrexia. Br. med. J. *ii:* 559 (1972).

20 European Malignant Hyperpyrexia Group: A protocol for the investigation of malignant hyperpyrexia (MH) susceptibility. Br. J. Anaesth. (in press, 1984).

21 Feinstein, M.B.: Inhibition of caffeine rigor and radiocalcium movements by local anaesthetics in frog sartorius muscle. J. gen. Physiol. *47:* 151–172 (1963).

22 Gallant; E.M.; Godt, R.E.; Gronert, G.A.: Role of plasma membrane defect in skeletal muscle in malignant hyperthermia. Muscle Nerve *2:* 491–494 (1979).

23 Gronert, G.A.; Heffron, J.A.; Taylor, S.R.: Skeletal muscle sarcoplasmic reticulum in porcine malignant hyperthermia. Eur. J. Pharmacol. *58:* 179–187 (1979).

24 Gronert, G.A.; Theye, R.A.: Halothane induced malignant hyperthermia: metabolic and haemodynamic changes. Anesthesiology *44:* 36 (1976).

25 Hall, G.M.; Lucke, J.N.; Orchard, C.; Lovell, R.; Lister, D.: Porcine malignant hyperthermia. VIII. Leg metabolism. Br. J. Anaesth. *54:* 941–947 (1982).

26 Halsall, P.J.; Ellis, F.R.: A screening test for the malignant hyperpyrexia phenotype using suxamethonium-induced contracture of muscle pretreated with caffeine and its inhalation by dantrolene. Br. J. Anaesth. *51:* 753–756 (1979).

27 Halsall, P.J.; Ellis, F.R.: The control of muscle contracture by the action of dantrolene on the sarcolemma. Acta anaesth. scand. *27:* 229–232 (1983).

28 Harriman, D.G.F.; Ellis, F.R.; Franks, A.J.; Summer, D.W.: Malignant hyperthermia myopathy in man – an investigation of 75 families; in Aldrete, Britt, 2nd Int. Symp. on Malignant Hyperthermia, p. 67 in Aldrete, Britt, (Grune & Stratton, New York 1978).

29 Isaacs, H.; Barlow, M.B.: The genetic background to malignant hyperpyrexia revealed by serum creatinine phosphokinase estimations in asymptomatic relatives. Br. J. Anaesth. *42:* 1077–84 (1970).

30 Isaacs, H.; Heffron, J.J.A.: Morphological and biochemical defects in muscles of human carriers of the malignant hyperthermia syndrome. Br. J. Anaesth. *47:* 475–481 (1975).

31 Kalow, W.; Britt, B.A.; Richter, A.: The caffeine test of isolated human muscle in relation to malignant hyperthermia. Can. Anaesth. Soc. J. *24:* 678–694 (1977).

32 Kalow, W.; Britt, B.A.; Terreau, M.E.; Haist, C.: Metabolic error of muscle metabolism after recovery from malignant hyperthermia. Lancet *ii:* 895 (1970).

33 Kerr, D.D.; Wingard, D.W.; Gatz, E.E.: Prevention of porcine malignant hyperthermia by epidural block. Anesthesiology *42:* 307–311 (1975).

34 Lister, D.; Hall, G.M.; Lucke, J.N.: Catecholamines in suxamethonium-induced hyperthermia in pigs. (Abstract). Br. J. Anaesth. *46:* 803 (1974).

35 Lister, D.; Hall, G.M.; Lucke, J.N.: Porcine malignant hyperthermia. III. Adrenergic blockade. Br. J. Anaesth. *48:* 297–304 (1976).

36 Lucke, J.N.; Dent, H.; Hall, G.M.; Lovell, R.; Lister, D.: The effects of bilateral adrenalectomy and pretreatment with bretylium on the halothane induced response. Br. J. Anaesth. *50:* 241–246 (1978).

37 Marjanen, L.A.; Denborough, M.A.: Adenylate kinase and malignant hyperpyrexia. Br. J. Anaesth. *54:* 949–952 (1982).

38 Mitchell, G.; Heffron, J.A.A.: Porcine stress syndromes. Adv. Food Res. *28:* 167–229 (1982).

39 Moulds, R.F.; Denborough, M.A.: Procaine in malignant hyperpyrexia. Br. med. J. *iV:* 526–528 (1972).

40 Nelson, T.E.: Excitation-contraction coupling: a common aetiological pathway for malignant hyperthermia muscle; in Aldrete, Britt, Malignant hyperthermia, p. 23 (Grune & Stratton, New York 1978).

41 Willner, J.H.; Ceni, C.G.; Wood, D.S.: High skeletal muscle adenylate cyclase in malignant hyperthermia. Soc. clin. Invest. *6:* 1119–1124 (1981).

42 Wilson, M.E.; Ellis, F.R.: Predicting malignant hyperpyrexia (Abstract). Br. J. Anaesth. *51:* 66 (1979).

43 Wingard, D.W.: Malignant hyperpyrexia. A human stress syndrome. Lancet *ii:* 1450 (1974).

P. Jane Halsall, MB, University Department of Anaesthesia, St. James' Hospital, Leeds LS9 7TF (England)

PAR. Pseudo-Allergic Reactions. Involvement of Drugs and Chemicals, vol. 4, pp. 138–180 (Karger, Basel 1985)

Immunologic Abnormalities Induced by *D*-Penicillamine

C.I. Edvard Smith, Lennart Hammarström

Department of Clinical Immunology, Huddinge University Hospital, Huddinge, and Department of Immunobiology, Wallenberglaboratory, Karolinska Institute, Stockholm, Sweden

Introduction

D-Penicillamine, dimethyl cysteine, is a low molecular weight substance (fig. 1) which, due to its chelating properties, was originally introduced as a treatment for Wilson's disease by *Walshe* [1] in 1956 (table I). It has now become firmly established in the treatment of a number of additional disorders (table I) [1–11]. The drug has also been investigated for beneficial effects in several other human disorders with variable results (table II) [12–32] and has further been used in the treatment of animal disease (table III) [33–43]. Apart from the suggested mechanism of penicillamine in the case of Wilson's disease, little is known about the underlying mechanism in other disorders [for review, see 9–11]. However, the immune system, collagen synthesis and metal ion metabolism have most frequently been suggested as important targets. Penicillamine is not only known to have beneficial effects, it has also been reported to cause a number of adverse reactions. Also, in this respect, the mechanism of action is to a large extent unknown. The side effects can be subdivided into two groups depending on whether the immune system is believed to be primarily involved or not. In this review, we will discuss some of the data concerning the effects of penicillamine on the immune apparatus.

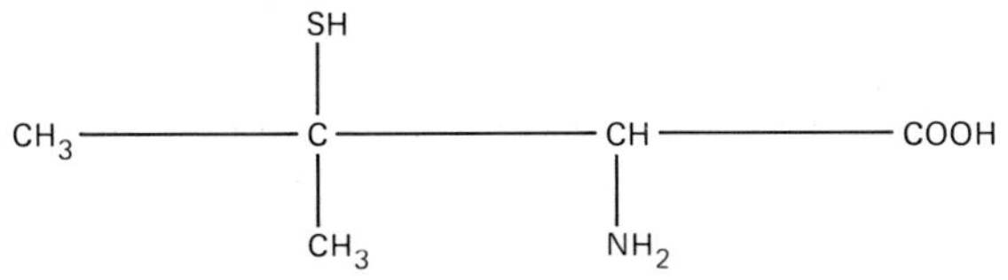

$$CH_3-\overset{\displaystyle SH}{\underset{\displaystyle CH_3}{C}}-\underset{\displaystyle NH_2}{CH}-COOH$$

Fig. 1. Penicillamine.

Chemical Properties

Penicillamine is an analogue to the naturally occurring amino acid, cysteine. In the early days of penicillamine treatment, a mixture of *D*(–) and *L*(+) forms were used, whereas today only the *D*(–) form is administered. Some symposia have been devoted to the analysis of the chemical properties of penicillamine and this has been discussed in detail [for reference, see 9–11]. The most reactive part of the penicillamine molecule is the thiol group. The thiol and the amino group have been proposed to be responsible for most of the biological properties. The chelating capacity of penicillamine seems to be mainly due to the thiol group, which binds metal ions through mercaptide formation. The complex of metal and penicillamine also has superoxide-dismutating activity and can act to decrease the number of free radicals. Furthermore, the thiol in penicillamine forms mixed disulphides via the interaction with sulph-hydryl- or disulphate-containing proteins. Penicillamine can also interact with aldehydes to form a thiazolidine ring. These latter interactions seem to be of importance for the interference with collagen cross-linking. In this interaction, the thiol as well as the amino group participates. The amino group also contributes to the binding of penicillamine to certain molecules such as DNA. Finally, the two methyl groups in penicillamine sterically interfere with the –SH group and can protect it from oxidization.

Adverse Reactions

Toxicity limits the usefulness of penicillamine in many patients. Adverse effects of the drug have been decreased by the use of lower daily doses [43–45] but still constitutes a major problem. The information concerning the role of the immune apparatus in these toxic phenomena is far from complete. Thus, to what extent immunologic reactions contribute

Table I. Diseases in which *D*-penicillamine is commonly used as a drug treatment

Disease	Report	Reference
Wilson's disease	*Walshe,* 1956	1
Lead poisoning	*Boulding and Baker,* 1957	2
Cystinuria	*Crawhall* et al., 1963	3
Rheumatoid arthritis	*Jaffe,* 1964	4
Progressive systemic sclerosis	*Harris and Sjoerdsma,* 1966	5
Chronic active hepatitis	*Alexander and Kludas,* 1969	6
Juvenile chronic arthritis	*Schairer and Stoeber,* 1976	7
Primary biliary cirrhosis	*Jain* et al., 1977	8

Table II. Diseases in which *D*-penicillamine has been investigated for beneficial affects

Disease	Report	Reference
Macroglobulinemia	*Block* et al. 1960	12
Haemolytic anemia	*Ritzmann and Levin,* 1961	13
Cadmium poisoning	*Holden,* 1966	14
Mercury poisoning	*Swensson and Ulfvarson,* 1967	15
Cryoglobulinemia	*Goldberg and Barnett,* 1970	16
Unilateral keratoconus	*François* et al., 1973	17
Morphea (localized cutaneous scleroderma)	*Moynahan,* 1973	18
Ankylosing spondylitis	*Golding,* 1974	19
Polymyositis	*Golding,* 1974	19
Osteoarthrosis	*Herbert* et al., 1974	20
Keloid	*Moynahan,* 1974	21
Neonatal hyperbilirubinemia	*Lakatos* et al., 1976	22
Psoriatic arthritis	*Recordier* et al., 1976	23
Duchenne muscular dystrophy	*Bradley* et al., 1977	24
Coalworker's pneumoconiosis	*Evans,* 1977	25
Arsenic poisoning	*Peterson and Rumack,* 1977	26
Sjögren's and Raynaud's syndrome	*Hay* et al., 1978	27
Amyloidosis	*Jaffe,* 1978	28
Felty's syndrome	*Jaffe,* 1978	28
Interstitial lung disease	*Goodman* et al., 1981	29
Eosinophilic granuloma	*Petherham* et al., 1981	30
Amyotrophic lateral sclerosis	*Conradi* et al., 1982	31
Generalized argyria	*Johansson* et al., 1982	32

Table III. D-Penicillamine treatment in animal diseases

Disorder	Species	Report	Reference
Adjuvant arthritis	rabbit	*Klamer* et al., 1968	33
Pertussis vaccine edema	rat	*Arrigoni-Martelli* et al., 1976	34
Hereditary avian muscular dystrophy	chicken	*Chou* et al., 1977	35
Chronic antigen-induced arthritis	rabbit	*Hunneyball* et al., 1977	36
Experimental amyloidosis	mouse	*Savage* et al., 1980	37
Seizure	baboon	*Alley* et al., 1981	38
Lupus syndrome	mouse	*Harris and Chandler,* 1981	39
Type-II collagen-induced polyarthritis	rat	*Kerwar* et al., 1981	40
Hepatoma growth	rat	*Tryfiates,* 1981	41
Experimental granulation tissue	rat	*Hølund* et al., 1982	42
Delayed hypersensitivity	guinea pig	*Honma and Nakayama,* 1982	43

Table IV. Common adverse reactions during penicillamine treatment

Adverse reaction	Reported frequency, %			
	Baum, 1979 [46] (n = 1,100)	*Kean* et al., 1980 [47] (n = 84)	*Stein* et al., 1980 [48] (n = 259)	*Dawkins* et al., 1981 [49] (n = 500)
Dysgeusia (altered taste)	13	12	20	8
Rash	12	32	44	16
Proteinuria	9	18	7	22
Gastrointestinal disturbance	7	8	18	10
Thrombocytopenia	7	17	3	13
Leukopenia	2	7	3	13
Stomatitis	2	4	10	8

to e.g. leukopenia and thrombocytopenia is still an open question. However, in a number of adverse reactions, the immune system is believed to be primarily involved. Thus, several patients with penicillamine-induced autoimmunity have been described. Table IV summarizes the findings in four reports [46–49] of the most common adverse reactions on a total of 2,000 penicillamine-treated individuals. Although the frequency figures vary somewhat between the different reports, rash, dysgeusia

Table V. Less common and uncommon adverse reactions during penicillamine treatment (reactions in which an association with the immune system has not been demonstrated)

Adverse reaction	Report/review	Reference
Less common reactions		
Bronchiolitis and bronchitis	*Epler* et al., 1979	50
Myelotoxicity	*Kay,* 1979	51
Mammary gigantism	*Rooney and Cleland,* 1981	52
Cholestasis and other hepatotoxic effects	*Seibold* et al., 1981	53
Pyridoxine deficiency (anemia, neuropathy)	*Pool* et al., 1981	54
	Sullivan et al., 1981	55
	Rothschild, 1982	56
Penicillamine dermopathy	*Levy* et al., 1983	57
Elastosis perforans seropigmentosa	*Levy* et al., 1983	57
Uncommon reactions		
Acute colitis	*Hickling and Fuller,* 1979	58
Yellow nail syndrome	*Lubach and Marghescu,* 1979	59
Hypertrichosis	*Munroe and Darley,* 1979	60
Pulmonary eosinophilia	*Davies and Lloyd Jones,* 1980	61
Pneumonitis	*Camus* et al., 1982	62
Acute lymphoblastic leukemia	*Gilman and Holtzman,* 1982	63
Gynecomastia	*Reid* et al., 1982	64
Cutis laxa	*Harpey* et al., 1983	65

(altered taste sensation), proteinuria and gastrointestinal disturbances dominate. Stomatitis, leukopenia and thrombocytopenia are also common side effects, followed by a number of reactions such as nausea, hot flashes, fever, polyarthralgias, cystitis and hematemesis [46–49]. The majority of toxic reactions occurred within the first 6 months but proteinuria and thrombocytopenia were more common in the 6- to 12-month treatment period. In most cases, the side effects disappeared during continued treatment. Even if the dose is often reduced when toxicity is observed, this is not a prerequisite for the disappearance of side effects. A number of less common adverse reactions have also been described (table V) [50–65]. In some of these reactions, the association with drug treatment seems to be clear. However, certain side effects are less well documented and merely represent possible adverse reactions. Data have been presented indicating that certain HLA–DR antigens exist in increased frequencies in patients treated with gold or penicillamine [66–68]. The observations with regard to penicillamine have not been confirmed by other researchers [69], and the original findings have also been re-evaluated and an effect of the sulphoxidation status has been suggested instead [70]. Conflicting reports have also been published concerning the influence of previous gold toxicity on subsequent development of penicillamine toxicity [71, 72].

Effects of Penicillamine on the Immune System

Penicillamine is used as a treatment in several diseases where immune mechanisms are supposed to play an important role. As already pointed out, the mechanism of the penicillamine effect in immunologic disorders is unknown. Several investigators have suggested immunosuppressive effects and, as will be presented, effects on B as well as T lymphocytes, macrophages and granulocytes have all been described. The original hypothesis advocating the use of penicillamine in the treatment of rheumatoid arthritis (RA) was the possibility that the drug would dissociate IgM molecules with rheumatoid factor activity. IgM rheumatoid factor is decreased, but the effect does not seem to be due to dissociation of the IgM molecule. Other immunoglobulin classes are also affected.

Penicillamine also causes a number of adverse reactions where effects on the immune system are believed to be of primary importance. Thus, several autoimmune phenomena have been described. However, as will be discussed, the autoimmune reactions do not seem to involve all types of autoimmunity but rather to be restricted to certain diseases.

Several basic questions can be asked concerning the possibility of a drug-induced disease. Does the idiopathic correspondence to the drug-induced disease occur at an increased frequency in the primary disease in the *absence* of the drug? If this is the case, is a true increment recorded or is it merely secondary to this spontaneous co-occurrence? Is the drug-induced disorder in all respects identical to the idiopathic form, or are there any differences? The most apparent evidence for penicillamine-induced autoimmunity, is the finding that discontinuation of the drug results in disappearance of the disease.

It is possible that basically different forms of even defined autoimmune disease entities exists and that the etiology differs. If this is the case, the penicillamine-induced form may only correspond to one of these subgroups.

Penicillamine-Induced Myasthenia gravis

More than 110 cases of myasthenia gravis have been reported in the literature during penicillamine treatment (table VI) [32, 33, 73–108]. As can be seen 104 (96%) were patients with RA, 2 had Wilson's disease (both of which were males) and only 1 patient each had systemic sclerosis and primary biliary cirrhosis, respectively. 74 females and 20 males (female:male ratio 3.7:1) were reported to develop this syndrome. The female:male ratio was 4.0:1 in the RA group. *Bucknall* et al. [109] reported a mean age of 48 and a mean duration of 10 months of penicillamine treatment before the development of myasthenia gravis. In the review of *Bucknall* et al. [109] 13 patients received a daily dose of 750 mg or more compared with 7 receiving a maximum of 500 mg daily. In the review by *Albers* et al. [92], the mean age of onset of myasthenia gravis in 39 females with RA on penicillamine treatment was 47 years as compared to 45 years in 6 men. As the authors point out, this contrasts to the reported mean age of onset of idiopathic myasthenia of 29 years for women and 35 years for men [110]. However, since the penicillamine-induced disease occurs already after less than a year of therapy, this probably merely reflects the age of the treated patients. In the review of *Albers* et al. [92], the mean duration after penicillamine treatment until myasthenia was 8 months. 26 patients had mild myasthenia and only 4 developed more severe symptoms. There was no evident relationship between the cumulative dosage and the severity of symptoms. *Albers* et al. [92] also report that in 32 of 45 published cases of penicillamine-induced myasthenia gravis, the symptoms completely disappeared after the drug was discontinued. In 4 cases the disease persisted. However, penicillamine does not only induce autoimmune *disease.* Thus, the mean serum acethylcholine receptor antibody titer in patients without myasthenia gravis has been reported to increase after drug treatment [for reference see 108].

Differences between Idiopathic and Drug-Induced Myasthenia

As previously outlined, one important question is whether there is an increased frequency of idiopathic myasthenia gravis in RA patients. It must be stated that 1–6.7% of patients with myasthenia gravis have RA [74, 109–111]. The possibility that this high frequency is related to the 'two-disease fallacy' concept must be kept in mind. The frequency of idiopathic myasthenia gravis in RA patients is not known. *Dawkins* et al. [113] have suggested a frequency of 1% of penicillamine-induced myasthenia, but could observe a frequency of only 0.2% (1 of 500) in their own material. A similar figure was obtained by *Sundström and Schuma* [91]: 0.25% (1 of 400). Due to the infrequent observations of idiopathic as well as drug-induced myasthenia gravis, any reliable frequency figures cannot be obtained at present. Racial differences may also exist.

However, the features of the drug-induced myasthenia seem to differ in several respects as compared with those of the idiopathic disease. Furthermore, as already mentioned, in the majority of cases there seems to be a kinetic relationship between penicillamine administration and disease. The similarities between the penicillamine-induced disorder and the idiopathic disease include electrophysiological signs and a positive response to edrophonium [73, 74], thymic abnormalities [76, 86] as well as the production of acethylcholine and muscle antibodies (table VI) [112–114]. However, the interspecies cross-reactivity of the acetylcholine receptor antibodies is higher in the idiopathic disorder as compared with that of the drug-induced form [115]. It has been suggested that this does not represent a true difference between the two disorders but merely depends on the length of the autoimmune stage [116]. This argument has not been settled and it is also debated whether the avidity of acetylcholine receptor antibodies is increased or decreased in the drug-induced form [116, 117]. Anti-striational antibodies have been reported to occur in as much as 20% of all RA patients treated with penicillamine and is mainly of the IgM type [113, 114]. On the other hand, anti-striational antibodies in the idiopathic disease are mainly IgG in origin [113], at least some of which belong to the IgG1 and IgG4 subclasses [118].

In only a few cases has the thymus been examined by histology in the drug-induced disease. Thymomas have not been observed, but thymic hyperplasia has been reported [76, 86]. Thymic hyperplasia has also been found after penicillamine treatment in the Rhesus monkey [119]. One important difference between the idiopathic disease and the drug-induced syndrome has recently been reported for HLA associations. Thus, in the spontaneous disease the frequency of the HLA-B8/Dw3/DR3 antigens is increased [120–122], whereas the antigens Bw35/DRI have an increased prevalence in the drug-induced disorder [106b, 107, 122]. These findings clearly argue in favor of the idea that drug-induced myasthenia gravis is a separate disease entity. However, it may well be that it corresponds to a subgroup of the idiopathic form.

Table VI. Penicillamine-induced myasthenia gravis

Report	Reference	Diagnosis	Number of cases	Sex	Positive test for acetylcholine receptor antibodies	HLA tissue typing
Miehlke and Jentsch, 1973	73	RA	1	–	–	–
Ott and Schmidt, 1974	74	RA	2	–	–	–
Bálint et al., 1975	75	RA	2	F	–	–
Bucknall et al., 1975	76	RA	4	F	–	–
Czlonkowska, 1975	77	Wilson's disease	1	M	–	–
Delrieu et al., 1975	78	RA	1	F	–	–
Dawkins et al., 1975	79	Wilson's disease	1	M	–	–
Schmidt and Kommerell, 1976	80	RA	1	F	–	–
Seitz et al., 1976	81	RA	12	F	–	–
Bucknall, 1977	82	RA	9	6 F	–	–
Gordon and Burnside, 1977	83	RA	1	F	–	–
Verret et al., 1977	84	RA	1	F	–	–
Verbraeken et al., 1978	85	RA	1	F	–	–
Rosenberger, 1978	86	RA (2)	5	1 F/1 M	–	–
Russell and Lindstrom, 1978	87	RA	3	F	+	+
Vincent et al., 1978	88	RA	3	2 F/1 M	+	+
Froelich et al., 1979	89	RA	1	F	–	–
Keesey and Novom, 1979	90	RA	1	F	+	+
Sundström and Schuma, 1979	91	RA	2	1 F/1 M	–	–
Albers et al., 1980	92	RA	1	F	+	+
Blanlœil et al., 1980	93	RA	1	F	–	–
Heyn, 1980	94	RA	2	F	–	–

Johansson et al., 1982	32	RA	1	–	–	–
Rosseau and Dieudonné, 1980	95	RA	1	F	–	–
Torres et al., 1980	96	systemic sclerosis	1	F	–	+
Bocanegra et al., 1981	97	RA	1	M	+	+
Lang et al., 1981	98	RA	2	M	+	+
Rodat et al., 1981	99	RA	2	F	–	+
Klamer et al., 1968	33	RA	1	M	–	–
Weinzierl et al., 1981	100	primary biliary cirrhosis	1	F	–	–
Wysocka et al., 1981	101	RA	2	1 F/1 M	–	–
Essigman, 1982	102	RA	1	M	+	–
Fawcett et al., 1982	103	RA	2	F	+	+
Gietka, 1982	104	RA	2	F	–	–
Vincent and Newson-Davis,, 1982[1]	105	RA	8	3 F/5 M	+	–
Woimant et al., 1982	106a	RA	1	F	+	+
Delamere et al., 1983	106b	RA	18	14 F/4 M	+	+
Garlepp et al., 1983[1]	107	RA	7	–	+	+
Smith et al., 1983	108	RA	4	3 F/1 M	+	+
		104 RA 2 Wilson's disease 1 primary biliary cirrhosis 1 systemic sclerosis	111	74 F/20 M		

[1] Cases possibly presented in earlier reports not included.

Mechanism of Penicillamine-Induced Myasthenia

The study of the autoimmune mechanism of penicillamine has been hampered because of the lack of experimental animal models. Thus, mouse and rat strains tested so far have not been susceptible to the myasthenia gravis-inducing effects of *D*-penicillamine [108, 123], although effects on autoimmunity have been observed [108]. However, an experimental disease has been induced in guinea pigs [124, 125]. If the features of this experimental disease are similar to the idiopathic disorder in humans, it would be of great interest. In one report signs of myasthenia were found to occur within 48 h after penicillamine administration [126]. No anti-acethylcholine-receptor antibodies were found. This indicates that penicillamine can directly interfere with muscular transmission, as has been suggested elsewhere [127].

Although the effect of penicillamine in the autoimmune disorder does not involve a direct effect of the drug on transmission, other possibilities exist. It has been demonstrated that penicillamine has a certain affinity for the acetylcholine receptor [128] and alterations of the receptor structure could result in immunization. Furthermore, direct activation of B lymphocytes by penicillamine could result in autoantibody synthesis. A direct effect on thymus cells could also result in autoimmunity. More detailed analyses of the possible mechanisms for the autoimmune reactions have been presented [108, 113].

Penicillamine-Induced Pemphigus Syndrome

Penicillamine has been reported to induce a pemphigus syndrome. 48 cases have recently been reviewed [130] and 14 additional cases in the literature are presented in table VII [27, 130–154]. As can be seen, 84% (43 of 51) had RA. Idiopathic myasthenia gravis and pemphigus have been previously reported to be associated [155–157]. The overall female:male ratio was 1.4:1, whereas the corresponding ratio in the group of patients with RA developing pemphigus was 1.5:1. This ratio differs ($p < 0.05$) from that of the drug-induced myasthenia gravis (table VI). In the review of *Santa Cruz* et al. [152], several features of this pemphigus syndrome were reported: the dosage of *D*-penicillamine varied from 250 to 1,000 mg/day and the mean duration of treatment before the onset of pemphigus was 13 months. 18 of 34 patients developed what was indistin-

Table VII. Penicillamine-induced pemphigus syndrome

Report	References	Disease	Number of patients	Sex
Yung and Hambrick, 1982 (review)	28, 120–149	RA	30	18 F/12 M
		Wilson's disease	1	M
		systemic sclerosis	1	F
		scleroderma	1	M
		morphea	1	F
		Sjögren's syndrome	1	F
		unclassified	11 (13)[1]	–
Marsden et al., 1977[2]	150	psoriasis	1	M
		RA	3	2 F/1 M
Kennedy et al., 1978	151	psoriasis	1	M
		RA	1	M
Santa Cruz et al., 1981	152	scleroderma	1	F
		RA	3	2 F/1 M
Barety et al., 1982	153	RA	2	F
Zone et al., 1982	154	RA	4	2 F/2 M
		43 RA 4 scleroderma 2 psoriasis 1 Sjögren's syndrome 1 Wilson's disease	62	30 F/21 M

[1] 2 of the unclassified cases were reported by *Santa Cruz* et al. [152].
[2] Cases not included in the review of *Yung and Hambrick* [130].

guishable from idiopathic pemphigus foliaceus, 5 pemphigus vulgaris and 4 pemphigus erythematosus. Furthermore the penicillamine-induced forms seemed to be more benign than the idiopathic form. Direct staining revealed deposits of antibodies (IgG) in the intercellular substance of the epidermis in 20 of 26 specimens. Intercellular deposits of autoantibodies were found in 18 of 28 patients as measured by indirect immunofluorescence using patient serum. Most cases resolved within a few months after cessation of the drug.

Intercellular epithelial antibodies have been found in myasthenia gravis patients in the absence of pemphigus and thymic abnormalities have been found in pemphigus in the absence of myasthenia gravis [158]. Furthermore, dermal-epidermal junction immunofluorescence staining, mainly of IgM type, has been reported in 23% (15 of 70) of RA patients [158]. Pemphigus occasionally occurs in patients with RA not being treated with *D*-penicillamine [159, 160]. However, as is the case with myasthenia gravis, any reliable frequency figures are to our knowledge not available at present.

Troy et al. [161] have reported a case of bullous pemphigoid and reviewed the differences between the idiopathic disease and the drug-induced disorder. They state that the drug-induced form differs in that it usually has a limited and localized cutaneous involvement and that oral involvement is rare (13%). They also reported that an immunofluorescence pattern indicative of pemphigus erythematosus occurs in 25% of the drug-induced form. This figure is somewhat higher than the figure of 4 in 28 having the erythematosus variant in the review of *Santa Cruz* et al. [152]. Based on in vitro experiments, the lesions in the penicillamine-induced pemphigus have been suggested to be caused directly by the effect of the drug on collagen synthesis and not via immune mechanisms [162]. The possible association to HLA-antigens has been reviewed by *Zone* et al. [154], who report 7 cases. HLA-B15 was detected in 5, an increase which, however, was not statistically significant. Idiopathic pemphigus has been reported to be associated with HLA-antigens [163–165]. The number of patients with penicillamine-induced pemphigus in which HLA antigens have been studied is too small to draw any conclusions concerning associations. In view of the interesting results obtained in drug-induced myasthenia gravis [107, 122], tissue typing of the pemphigus patients is warranted.

Penicillamine-Induced Polymyositis

Penicillamine has been reported to induce polymyositis in 16 cases (table VIII) [102, 166–179]. 14 cases were previously reviewed by *Doyle* et al. [166]. 14 patients (88%) had RA, 1 systemic sclerosis and 1 Wilson's disease. The frequency of RA was not significantly different from that found in penicillamine-induced pemphigus or myasthenia gravis, but the polymyositis material was small. The female:male ratio was 3:1 in the total material and 3.6:1 in the RA group of patients. The dosage of *D*-penicillamine ranged from 250 to 1,200 mg/day and the mean duration of

Table VIII. Penicillamine-induced polymyositis

Report	References	Disease	Number of cases	Sex
Doyle et al., 1983 (review)	166–178	RA	12	11 F/1 M
		Wilson's disease	1	F
		systemic sclerosis	1	M
Fisher and Pennebaker, 1981	179	RA	1	M
Essigman, 1982	102	RA	1	M
		14 RA 1 Wilson's disease 1 systemic sclerosis	16	12 F/4 M

treatment before the onset of polymyositis was 9 months. Most cases resolved within a few months after cessation of drug therapy. In spite of the fact that penicillamine can induce polymyositis, it has also been used as a treatment in polymyositis (table II) [19]. *Doyle* et al. [166] reviewed 2 and reported 1 case of *D*-penicillamine-induced cardiac disease. Although clinical myocaridal involvement is seen in idiopathic polymyositis, it is relatively uncommon and usually mild [180]. Idiopathic polymyositis, like pemphigus, has been reported in several patients with myasthenia gravis [155, 181]. As previously outlined in the pemphigus section, HLA tissue typing would be similarily warranted in penicillamine-induced polymyositis patients. An association with HLA-B8 has been reported in the idiopathic disorder [182].

Penicillamine-Induced Lupus Erythematosus

25 patients with penicillamine-induced lupus erythematosus are presented in table IX [102, 183–194]. 15 (60%) had RA, 8 (32%) had Wilson's disease and 2 had cystinuria. This percentage is significantly lower as compared with the 96% of the patients with myasthenia gravis induced by *D*-penicillamine having RA ($p < 0.001$). Most cases resolved within a few months after cessation of therapy. The female: male ratio in the total material was 4.8:1 and in the RA group 7.5:1. The dose of penicillamine was

Table IX. Penicillamine-induced lupus erythematosus

Report	Reference	Disease	Number of patients	Sex	Dose of penicillamine	
					< 1 g	≥ 1 g
Boudin et al., 1971	183	Wilson's disease	1	F		1
Caille et al., 1971	184	Wilson's disease	1	F		1
Harpey et al., 1971	185	Wilson's disease	1	F		1
Rasmussen, 1971	186	cystinuria	1	M		1
Oliver et al, 1972	187	cystinuria	1	F		1
Appelboom et al., 1978	188	Wilson's disease	1	F		1
Rimbaud et al., 1973	189	RA	2	F		2
Crozet et al., 1974	190	RA	1	F		1
Harkcom et al., 1978	191	RA	1	F	1	
Kirby et al., 1979	192	RA	4	3 F/1 M	–	–
Walshe, 1981	193	Wilson's disease	4	1 F/1 M	–	–
Chalmers et al., 1982	194	RA	6	F	5	1
Essigman, 1982	102	RA	1	M	1	
		15 RA 8 Wilson's disease 2 cystinuria	25	19 F/4 M	7	10

≥ 1 g in 10 of 17 reported patients. Since a high-dose regimen is used in Wilson's disease, it is not clear whether this disease itself or the dose regimen is primarily associated with the induction of a lupus erythematosus syndrome. However, the doses used in patients developing the lupus erythematosus syndrome are high as compared with those used in patients developing, e.g., myasthenia gravis or pemphigus after *D*-penicillamine treatment. The mean duration of treatment before onset of lupus erythematosus symptoms was 22 months, based on calculations using data from 17 reported patients. However, *Walshe* [193] has reported 2 extreme cases with Wilson's disease where 1 developed lupus erythematosus after 2 weeks of penicillamine treatment and 1 after 20 years. If these 2 patients are included the mean duration time increases to 35 months. 22 months is a longer induction phase as compared to myasthenia gravis, pemphigus and polymyositis. However, it is possible that certain disorders are more easily diagnosed at an earlier stage than others and, although unlikely, it could be argued that this is the reason for the time differences observed.

The frequency of penicillamine-induced lupus erythematosus has been estimated to be 0.4–2% [113, 194] in patients with RA. In patients with Wilson's disease, 'serological changes typical for lupus erythematosus' were found in 7% and clinical lupus erythematosus in 3% [193]. If one compares these frequency estimations with the number of reported patients in the literature, irrespective of the fact that we in no way claim that we have found all reports, the number is low. In myasthenia gravis where a lower incidence has been found [91, 113], the number of reported cases is much higher. The reason for this is not known and the co-occurrence of idiopathic RA and lupus erythematosus is uncommon [195]. One possible reason could be that anti-nuclear antibodies are being monitored and that penicillamine treatment is discontinued if these antibodies appear. Anti-nuclear antibodies may develop in asymptomatic patients during the course of therapy [196]. Furthermore, it is evident that some of the clinical manifestations of RA are also found in lupus erythematosus. In contrast to lupus erythematosus induced by several other drugs [197], the pencillamine-induced cases have antibodies directed against double-stranded DNA [192]. In one of the reports [194], all 6 patients with penicillamine-induced lupus erythematosus were examined for HLA antigens. However, more patients are needed in order to see any possible differences as compared with idiopathic lupus erythematosus. Interestingly, however, none of the 6 patients had HLA-B8 DR3, antigens which are associated with the spontaneous form [198].

Penicillamine-Induced Goodpasture's Syndrome

Penicillamine has been reported as the cause of Goodpasture's syndrome in 9 cases (table X) [199–205]. 5 patients (56%) had RA 3 had Wilson's disease and 1 primary biliary cirrhosis. The female:male ratio in the total group was 1.3:1. The dose of penicillamine was $\geq$ 1 g in 7 of the reported patients. Thus, it seems as if a high dose increases the risk for the development of Goodpasture's syndrome. As in drug-induced lupus erythematosus, the frequency of Wilson's disease patients was high. Whether this reflects the dose regimen or is due to Wilson's disease in itself is not known. The mean duration of treatment before onset of Goodpasture's syndrome was 35 (7–84) months, based on calculations using data

Table X. Penicillamine-induced Goodpasture's syndrome

Report	Reference	Disease	Number of patients	Sex	Dose of penicillamine	
					<1 g	≥1 g
Sternlieb et al., 1976	199	Wilson's disease	3	2 F/1 M		3
Gibson et al., 1976	200	RA	1	M		1
McCormick et al., 1976	201	RA	1	M		1
Matloff and Kaplan, 1980	202	primary biliary cirrhosis	1	F		1
Gavaghan et al., 1981	203	RA	1	M	1	
Hasselman et al., 1982	204	RA	1	F	1	
Swainson et al., 1982	205	RA	1	F		1
		5 RA 3 Wilson's disease 1 primary biliary cirrhosis	9	5 F/4 M	2	7

from the reported 8 patients. Only 2 patients [201, 205] had a therapy duration of less than 2 years. Thus, it is clear that the inductive phase in Goodpasture's syndrome is much longer than in other penicillamine-induced autoimmune disorders (myasthenia gravis, pemphigus, polymyositis and possibly even lupus erythematosus). There is one clear difference between the penicillamine-induced disorder and the idiopathic form. Thus, anti-glomerular basement membrane antibodies have not been reported in the drug-induced disease. 1 patient with the drug-induced disorder was investigated for HLA antigens [203]. He was found not to have the HLA-DR2 antigen, which has been reported in increased frequency in patients with idiopathic Goodpasture's syndrome [206].

Penicillamine has also been reported to induce nephropathy in the absence of Goodpasture's syndrome [for review see 207]. As can be seen in table IV, proteinuria is one of the most common side effects of penicillamine treatment and it has been reported to occur more often in patients with RA or cystinuria than in those with Wilson's disease [208]. The dose and the speed of dose increments are of importance [207]. Histological examinations have revealed minimal changes, mesangioproliferative or membraneous nephropathy as well as progressive glomerulonephritis with crescent formation. The ultrastructural findings are those of an immune complex nephritis with subepithelial dense deposits [207]. Circulating immune complexes could be involved in the disease process and the amount of circulating immune complexes has indeed been reported to decrease after penicillamine treatment [209, 210].

Penicillamine and Lichen planus

Lichen planus has been reported in 25 patients treated with penicillamine (table XI) [211–214]. 24 of these had primary biliary cirrhosis and 1 patient had RA. However, 12 cases unrelated to penicillamine therapy were also observed in patients with primary biliary cirrhosis (table XI), clearly demonstrating an association between the two disorders. Penicillamine has also been reported to cause marked exacerbation of lichen planus in primary biliary cirrhosis patients [215]. The average duration after penicillamine treatment before onset of lichen planus was 11 months [214].

Idiopathic lichen planus has also been reported in patients with idiopathic myasthenia gravis [216–218], another of the disorders which can be induced by *D*-penicillamine. In spite of the fact that this might argue in favor of a drug-induced form also of lichen planus, little is known about the disease mechanism in the idiopathic form. However, an immunologic disturbance has been postulated and the disorder seems to occur in an increased frequency in patients with hypogammaglobulinemia [219]. It is possible that HLA-A3 is increased in the idiopathic form [220, 221], but analysis of DR antigens is warranted. Tissue typing of cells from patients with the penicillamine-induced form is in progress [214]. In conclusion, several findings argue in favor of a penicillamine-induced form of lichen planus, but since an association between the idiopathic forms of lichen planus and primary biliary cirrhosis do exist, additional information is needed until it can be established that penicillamine may induce lichen planus.

Multiple Autoimmunity and Rare Autoimmunity during Penicillamine Treatment

At least 2 patients have been reported to have developed more than one autoimmune disease during penicillamine treatment. *Delrieu* et al.

Table XI. Penicillamine and lichen planus

Report	Reference	Disease	Cases related to therapy with penicillamine	Cases not related to therapy with penicillamine
Van de Staak et al., 1975	211	RA	1	0
Seehafer et al., 1981	212	primary biliary cirrhosis	6	1
Graham-Brown et al., 1982	213	primary biliary cirrhosis	1	4
Powell et al., 1982	214	primary biliary cirrhosis	17	7
			24 primary bilary cirrhosis 1 RA	12 primary bilary cirrhosis

[78] reported a female with RA who developed myasthenia gravis and autoimmune thyroiditis. Myasthenia gravis occurred 14 months after the initiation of treatment and thyroiditis was found 10 months later. Penicillamine was discontinued when myasthenia gravis was diagnosed, but was reintroduced in a lower dose after 3 months. *Essigman* [102] reported a male with RA who developed lupus erythematosus, polymyositis and myasthenia gravis. Lupus erythematosus was diagnosed 6 years after the initiation of treatment and a few weeks later myasthenia gravis and polymyositis were observed.

Except for myasthenia gravis, pemphigus, polymyositis, lupus erythematosus, Goodpasture's disease and lichen planus, only a few cases of other autoimmune disorders have been reported after penicillamine treatment. However, it may well be that some of the less common adverse reactions listed in table V, such as e.g. bronchiolitis, are autoimmune in origin. Apart from the thyroiditis described above, another case has been presented by *Bertrand* et al. [222]. The patient was a female with primary biliary cirrhosis who, after 19 months of penicillamine treatment, developed an autoimmune thyroiditis. In 2 patients, thrombotic thrombocytopenic purpura has been reported. In a female with Wilson's disease, the symptoms appeared after 1 month [223] and in a female with RA symptoms also appeared after 1 month of penicillamine treatment [224]. Whether autoimmunity is involved in the mechanism of thrombocytopenic purpura is not known, and the short period of drug treatment might argue against this possibility. Sjörgren's syndrome has been reported in a female with RA being on penicillamine treatment for 6–8 weeks [225]. The authors also present 2 other possible cases. However, patients with Sjögren's syndrome have also been receiving penicillamine as a *treatment* [27]. Furthermore, in the case of thyroiditis and Sjögren's syndrome, it should be emphasized that these disorders normally co-exist with primary biliary cirrhosis and rheumatoid arthritis.

Effect of Penicillamine on Immunoglobulins

The original hypothesis when penicillamine was introduced as a treatment for RA was that the drug would reduce IgM molecules leading to the disappearance of immunoglobulins with rheumatoid factor activity [4]. This is no longer recognized as the mechanism of action [226], since sufficiently high concentrations are not found in vivo [227]. However, penicillamine treatment does result in a decrease of IgM [228, 229], but not IgG [229] rheumatoid factor levels. Furthermore, immune complexes have been reported to disappear in patients with RA [210] and primary biliary cirrhosis [209]. IgE has been reported to increase initially [230] whereas consistent changes of total IgM and IgG normally are not seen in either RA [229], cystinuria [231] or in Wilson's disease [232].

Effect of Penicillamine on IgA

As can be seen in table XII, 7 patients have been reported to develop IgA deficiency during penicillamine treatment [188, 210, 233–237]. 4 patients (57%) had Wilson's disease, 2 had RA and 1 had chronic active hepatitis. All were females and all had received a dose of penicillamine corresponding to $\geq$ 1 g/day. The mean duration of treatment before decreased IgA levels were detected was 14 (4–30) months, based on calculations from the 6 reported cases. IgA normally increased after cessation of treatment, but in some patients it remained low. There was no correlation between the serum IgA levels, the presence of secretory IgA and the frequency of infections (table XII). However, the material is too small to draw any conclusions concerning IgA levels and the frequency of infections.

Table XII. Penicillamine-induced IgA deficiency

Report	Reference	Disease	Number of patients	Sex	Dose g	Infections	IgA in serum g/l	Secretory IgA
Rimbaud et al., 1973	189	Wilson's disease	1	F	$\geqslant 1$	increased	0.13	–
Proesmans et al., 1976	233	Wilson's disease	1	F	$\geqslant 1$	increased	<0.1	absent
Hjalmarson et al., 1977	234	Wilson's disease	1	F	$\geqslant 1$	–	0.075	–
Michel et al., 1977	235	Wilson's disease	1	F	$\geqslant 1$	unchanged	<0.01	absent
Stanworth et al. 1977	236	RA	1	F	$\geqslant 1$	increased	0.070	absent
Götze, 1979	237	chronic active hepatitis	1	F	<1[1]	–	0.05	absent
Norberg et al., 1980	210	RA	1	–	–	–	0.1	–
		4 Wilson's disease 2 RA 1 chronic active hepatitis	7	6 F				

[1] The patient was a 6-year-old girl and was treated with 700 mg *D*-penicillamine/day. If body weight is taken into consideration she would probably be classified as >1 g.

There are three reports in which IgA deficiency in penicillamine treatment has been studied with regard to histocompatibility antigens [238–240]. However, the definition of IgA deficiency in two of these studies were < 0.8 and < 0.4 g/l, respectively. It may well be that this definition could be useful in certain circumstances, but it can hardly be used as an upper limit for IgA deficiency. In one of these reports, the possibility of an association between clinical response in RA and decreased levels of IgA is suggested [242]. However, at least 1 RA patient lacking IgA before treatment and still responding favorably to penicillamine has been described [240]. We have recently studied the HLA antigens [241] in the patient reported by *Hjalmarson* et al. [234]. This patient had A2; B18; 40; Cw3; DR4,7. An increased frequency of A2 has been noted in diphenylhydantoin-induced IgA deficiency [242]. However, in healthy individuals with the idiopathic form of IgA deficiency, an increased frequency of HLA-B8/DR3 has been demonstrated [243]. The mechanism underlying the induction of IgA deficiency remains unknown. However, it is possible that autoimmune mechanisms could be responsible for some of the idiopathic forms of IgA deficiency [244] and it is possible that this is also seen in the drug-induced disorder. Should this be the case, the patient reported by *Rimbaud* et al. [189] could also be included as a multiple autoimmunity case, since she also had penicillamine-induced lupus erythematosus.

Effects of Penicillamine on the Complement System

Strickland and Leu [232] studied C3 levels in 16 patients with Wilson's disease on penicillamine treatment. Complement levels were not greatly altered in any patient, although 3 had slight reductions. *Bacon* et al. [245] have reported that C3 and C4 levels were not changed significantly in RA patients during penicillamine administration. *Chwalinska-Sadowska and Baum* [246] reported a small reduction of the CH_{50} obtained at the highest concentrations used, 50 mg/ml (2.7 mmol) in in vitro experiments. *Mellbye and Munthe* [247] using higher concentrations (200 mmol) could completely abolish the CH_{50} activity. However, although the peak levels of penicillamine were possibly very high in occasional patients, these authors found no in vivo effect on CH_{50} in RA patients treated with 1,000 mg/day. In conclusion, no in vivo effects of penicillamine on the complement system have been found.

Effects of Penicillamine on T and B Lymphocytes

A number of investigators have studied the effects of penicillamine on T and B lymphocytes (table XIII) [34, 43, 103, 108, 248–260]. As is indicated in the table, in the earliest reports a mixture of *D*(–)- and *L*(+)-penicillamine was used. In the majority of reports, T-lymphocyte responses were decreased after penicillamine exposure. However, the process of T-lymphocyte activation is complex and involves, e.g., the participation of macrophages, and only few investigators have simultaneously studied accessory cells and T cells [255, 261]. Of the T-cell subsets, helper cells were reported to be inhibited [260]. However, other subsets have not been carefully investigated. In vivo antibody synthesis could be enhanced or inhibited depending on the time when penicillamine was given [248, 249]. *D*-penicillamine was also found to be mitogenic for B lymphocytes [108, 256]. In the majority of reports, autoimmunity was not studied, but in one report an increased production of autoantibodies in mice was detected [108].

Effects of Penicillamine on Macrophages and Granulocytes

Table XIV [255, 261–265] and table XV [246, 266–268] summarize the reported penicillamine-induced effects on macrophages and granulocytes. The macrophages studied [261, 263] showed an enhanced functional activity, whereas other investigators have been unable to observe such an effect [255]. Chemotaxis seems to be enhanced after in vivo treatment [266, 267], whereas addition of penicillamine in in vitro systems had an inhibitory effect [246, 267]. Two factors may be responsible for this discrepancy. In the in vivo experiments, there was a long-lasting exposure to penicillamine as compared to the situation in vitro. Moreover, the concentrations of pencillamine obtained in vitro, might be higher than those found in vivo.

Concluding Remarks

In this review, we have focussed on the immunologic abnormalities induced by *D*-penicillamine. Certain distinct disease patterns seem to exist. One group of disorders consists of myasthenia gravis, pemphigus and polymyositis. In the majority of these cases, they appeared within 1 year of treatment and were not dependent on high doses of penicillamine being administered. Furthermore, in most of these cases RA was the cause of the drug being instituted as treatment. In addition, an increased frequency of co-existence of these three diseases has been observed in the *absence* of penicillamine treatment. However, HLA studies have clearly demonstrated that different genetic markers are involved, at least in the penicillamine-induced as compared to the idiopathic form of myasthenia gravis.

What could then be the common denominator in these three disorders? One interesting observation is the occurrence of thymic abnormalities in idiopathic pemphigus in the absence of myasthenia gravis. Thymic abnormalities are certainly common in the idiopathic form of myasthenia gravis, but have also been observed in the penicillamine-induced disorder. Thus, although we have little direct evidence, it could be hypothesized that the thymus plays an important role in the disease process for all these three disorders, even if cells of the T-cell lineage are not necessarily the origin. In the drug-induced disorder cessation of penicillamine administration results in the disappearance of the autoimmune disease. However, if the thymus is of central importance in the idiopathic as well as in the drug-induced forms of these disease, it suggests that thymectomy might be of benefit not only in idiopathic myasthenia gravis but in autoimmune forms of pemphigus and polymyositis as well[1].

Another group of diseases induced by *D*-penicillamine is formed by lupus erythematosus and Goodpasture's syndrome. The penicillamine-induced form of these disorders differed from the previous group in several respects. There was a longer duration period between the beginning of treatment and onset of symptoms, the dose was higher and the percentage of RA as a cause of treatment was decreased. The latter finding could possibly reflect the dose regimen. Drug-induced Goodpasture's syndrome clearly differed from the idiopathic form in that not a single patient was reported to have antibodies directed against glomerular basement membrane.

Recent studies have indicated a possible association between penicillamine and lichen planus in primary biliary cirrhosis. Whether

[1] We have recently put forward this theory [*Smith, C.I.E.; Hammarström, L.* in Lancet *i:* 627, 1984] and in the same issue benefit from thymectomy in patients with polymyositis was reported [*Lane, R.J.M.; Hudgson, P.* in Lancet *i:* 626, 1984].

Table XIII. Effect of penicillamine on lymphocytes

Report	Reference	Type of penicillamine	Species	In vivo	In vitro	Effects (direct or indirect) on T cells	Effects (direct or indirect) on B cells	Effect of penicillamine
Tobin and Altman, 1964	248	*DL*	rabbit	+	–	+	+	increased antibody response if given 28 days before the antigen, human serum albumin
Altman and Tobin, 1965	249	*DL*	rabbit	+	–	+	+	decreased antibody response if given 1 day before the antigen, human serum albumin
Assem and Vickers, 1974	250	penicilline	human	+	–	+	+	penicilline allergy induces antibodies to penicillamine
Roath and Wills, 1974	251	*DL*	human	–	+	+	–	decreased phythemagglutinin induced ^{3}H-thymidine incorporation
Brandt and Svensson, 1975	252	*D*	human	+	–	+	+	decreased T (E rosettes) and non-T cells and increased granulocytes
Schumacher et al., 1975	253	*D*	human	–	+	+	–	decreased phythemagglutinin and mixed leukocyte reaction induced ^{3}H-thymidine incorporation
Arrigoni-Martelli et al., 1976	34	*D*	rat	+	–	+	–	enhanced delayed hypersensitivity to pertussis vaccine
Kendall and Hutchins, 1978	254	*D*	mouse	–	+	+	–	increased concanavalin A and mixed leucocyte reaction induced ^{3}H-thymidine incorporation initially; lacked mitogenicity; decreased *L*-cysteine levels resulting in nutrient deficiency

Lipsky and Ziff, 1978	255	*D*	human	–	+	+	–	inhibited the phythemagglutinin, concanavalin A and pokeweed mitogen induced ^{3}H-thymidine incorporation; $CuSO_4$ acted synergistically
Claesson et al., 1979	256	*D*	mouse rat human	–	+	+	+	mitogenic for mouse, rat and human spleen cells; activated mouse spleen B and human spleen T cells
Kosaka, 1979	257	*D*	human	+	–	+	+	increased peripheral blood T cells and decreased B cells
Room et al., 1979	258	*D*	human	–	+	+	–	decreased phythemagglutinin induced ^{3}H-thymidine incorporation; *L*-cysteine abolished the effect; $CuSO_4$ acted synergistically
Feickert and Schumacher, 1980	259	*D*	human	–	+	+	–	inhibited phythemagglutinin induced ^{3}H-thymidine incorporation by an effect on the cell membrane
Lipsky and Ziff, 1980	260	*D*	human	–	+	+	+	inhibited T-helper cells for B lymphocytes; no direct effect on B lymphocytes
Fawcett et al., 1982	103	*D*	human	–	+	+	+	increased polyclonal as well as acetylcholine receptor antibodies after pokeweed mitogen stimulation
Honma and Nakayama, 1982	43	*D*	guinea pig	+	–	+	–	enhanced delayed hypersensitivity to ferritin
Smith et al., 1983	108	*D*	mouse human	+	+	+	+	mitogenic for mouse spleen B cells and weakly for human peripheral blood lymphocytes; increased autoantibody formation in mice

Table XIV. Effect of penicillamine on macrophages

Report	Reference	Type of penicillamine	Species	In vivo	In vitro	Effect of penicillamine
Binderup et al., 1978	261	*D*	rat	–	+	enhanced the functional activity of macrophages in the lymphocyte response to concanavalin A
Lipsky and Ziff, 1978	255	*D*	human	–	+	did not alter the accessory cell capacity of monocytes in the T-lymphocyte response to concanavalin A or to pokeweed mitogen
Binderup and Arrigoni-Martelli, 1979	262	*D*	rat	–	+	was bound firmly to macrophages; entered and diffused freely out of lymphocytes
Binderup et al., 1980	263	*D*	rat	+	–	same result as in *Binderup* et al. [261]
Binderup et al., 1980	264	*D*	rat	+	+	preincubation increased the macrophage uptake of aggregated human γ-globulin
De Vries et al., 1982	265	*D*	human	–	+	lymphocytes as compared to macrophages were more sensitive to toxic effects of penicillamine; induced stimulatory as well as inhibitory effects on the pokeweed mitogen-induced response

Table XV. Effect of penicillamine on granulocytes

Report	Reference	Type of penicillamine	Species	In vivo	In vitro	Effect of penicillamine
Chwalinska-Sadowska and Baum, 1976	246	*D*	human	–	+	decreased chemotaxis, while phagocytosis and lysosomal enzyme release was unaffected
Cunningham et al., 1978	266	*D*	rat	+	+	increased leucocyte migration in vivo; no effect on chemotaxis or random migration in vitro
Mowat, 1978	267	*D*	human	+	+	decreased or no effect on chemotaxis or random migration in vitro; improved chemotaxis after in vivo treatment
Meacock et al., 1981	268	*D*	rat	+	–	no effect on chemotaxis

this is secondary to a primary association of the idiopathic forms can not at present be resolved. However, a primary association between penicillamine administration and the subsequent development of IgA deficiency seems established. In this form of immunoglobulin deficiency, a high-dose regimen seems to be crucial. This could be indicative of toxicity, but the idea of an autoimmune effect is equally attractive to us.

Penicillamine treatment can result in the occurrence of certain types of 'autoimmune' (autoallergic) diseases. Little is known about the pathomechanism of these adverse reactions to penicillamine. However, the available evidence argues in favour of a reaction not directed against penicillamine itself. Thus, these processes might be referred to as pseudo-allergic reactions.

Acknowledgements

Part of the work presented in this review was supported by the Swedish Medical Research Council, the MS Foundation, the Walter, Ellen and Lennart Hesselman Foundation and the Fredrik and Ingrid Thuring Foundation. We would like to express our sincere gratitude to the staff at the Huddinge University Hospital Library and the Karolinska Institute Library for their kind help in obtaining references and to Ms *Gunilla Tillinger* and *Lena Carlson* for excellent typing.

References

1 Walshe, J.M.: Penicillamine: a new oral therapy for Wilson's disease. Am. J. Med. *2:* 487–495 (1956).

2 Boulding, J.E.; Baker, R.A.: Treatment of metal poisoning with penicillamine. Lancet *i:* 985 (1957).

3 Crawhall, J.C.; Scowen, E.F.; Watts, R.W.E.: Effect of penicillamine on cystinuria. Br. med. J. *i:* 588–590 (1963).

4 Jaffe, I.A.: Rheumatoid arthritis with arteritis: report of a case treated with penicillamine. Ann. Intern. Med. *61:* 556–563 (1964).

5 Harris, E.D.; Sjoerdsma, A.: Effect of penicillamine on human collagen and possible application to treatment of scleroderma. Lancet *ii:* 996–999 (1966).

6 Alexander, M.; Kludas, M.: Kollagensynthese – Hemmung durch *D*-Penicillamine bei chronisch aggressiver Hepatitis. Münch med. Wschr. 111: 847–850 (1969).

7 Schairer, H.; Stoeber, E.: Long-term follow-up of 235 cases of juvenile rheumatoid arthritis treated with *D*-penicillamine; in Munthe, Penicillamine research in rheumatoid disease, pp. 279–281 (Fabritius and Sønner, Oslo 1976).

8 Jain, S.; Scheuer, P.J.; Samourian, S.; McGee, J.O.D.; Sherlock, S.: A controlled trial of *D*-penicillamine therapy in primary biliary cirrhosis. Lancet *i:* 831–834 (1977).

9 Feltkamp, T.E.W: Fundamental studies on pencillamine for rheumatoid diseases. Scand. J. Rheumatol., suppl. 28, pp. 1–110 (1979).

10 Proceedings of the International Symposium on Penicillamine. J. Rheumatol. 8: suppl. 7, pp. 1–181 (1981).

11 Maini, R.N.; Berry, H.: Modulation of autoimmunity and disease. The penicillamine experience (Praeger, New York 1981).

12 Block, M.S.; Prasad, A.; Anastasi, A.; Brigs, B.R.: Serum protein changes in Waldenstrom's macroglobulinemia during administration of a low molecular weight thiol (penicillamine) J. Lab. clin. Med. *56:* 212–217 (1960).

13 Ritzmann, S.E.; Levin, W.C.: Effect of mercaptanes in cold agglutination disease. J. Lab. clin. Med. *57:* 718–732 (1961).

14 Holden, H.: The use of penicillamine in cadmium-fume poisoning. Proc. 15th Int. Congr. Occup. Health, vol. 3, pp. 277–279 (1966).

15 Swensson, A.; Ulfvarson, U.: Experiments with different antidotes in acute poisoning by different mercury compounds. Int. Arch. Arbeitsmed. *24:* 12–50 (1967).

16 Goldberg, L.S.; Barnett, E.V.: Essential cryoglobulinemia. Immunologic studies before and after penicillamine. Archs intern. Med. *125:* 145–150 (1970).

17 François, J.; Cambie, E.; Feher, J.: Collagenase inhibition with penicillamine. Case report. Ophthalmologica, Basel *166:* 222–225 (1973).

18 Moynahan, E.J.: Morphea (localized cutaneous scleroderma) treated with low-dosage penicillamine (4 cases including coup de sabre) Proc. R. Soc. Med. *66:* 1083–1084 (1973).

19 Golding, D.N.: *D*-Penicillamine in ankylosing spondylitis and polymyositis. Post-grad med. J., suppl., pp. 62–64 (1974).

20 Herbert, C.M.; Jayson, M.I.V.; Lindberg, K.A.; Bailey, A.J.: The action of *D*-Penicillamine on collagen in scleroderma and osteo-arthrosis. Post-grad med. J., suppl., pp. 27–30 (1974).

21 Moynahan, E.J.: Penicillamine in the treatment of morphoea and keloid in children. Post-grad med. J. *50:* suppl. 2, pp. 39–40 (1974).

22 Lakatos, L.; Kövér, B.; Oroszlán, G.; Vekerdy, Z.: *D*-Penicillamine therapy in AB0 hemolytic disease of the newborn infant. Eur. J. Pediat. *123:* 133–135 (1976).

23 Recordier, A.-M.; Roux, H.; Mercier, P.; Maestracci, D.; Schiano, A.: A propos d'anomalies immunologiques au cours de traitement par penicillamine. Annls Méd. Int. *129:* 566–570 (1976).

24 Bradley, W.G.; Enomoto, A.; Gardner-Medwin, D.: A double-blind controlled trial of penicillamine therapy in Duchenne muscular dystrophy – interim comments. Proc. R. Soc. Med. *70:* suppl. 3, p. 94 (1977).

25 Evans, P.H.: Serum sulph-hydryl changes in rheumatoid coalworker's pneumoconiosis patients treated with *D*-penicillamine. Proc. R. Soc. Med. *70:* suppl. 3, pp. 95–97 (1977).

26 Peterson, R.G.; Rumack, B.H.: *D*-Penicillamine therapy of acute arsenic poisoning. J. Pediat. *91:* 661–666 (1977).

27 Hay, K.D.; Muller, H.K.; Reade, P.C.: *D*-Penicillamine-induced mucocutaneous lesions with features of pemphigus. Oral Surg. *45:* 385–395 (1978).

28 Jaffe, I.A.: *D*-Penicillamine. Bull. rheum. Dis. *28:* 948–952 (1978).

29 Goodman, M.; Knight, R.K.; Turner-Warwick, M.: Pilot study of penicillamine therapy in steroid failure patients with interstitial lung disease; in Maini, Berry, Modulation of autoimmunity and disease, pp. 291–299 (Praeger, New York 1981).

30 Petherham, I.S.; Holmes, P.; Turner-Warwick, M.: Penicillamine in eosinophilic granuloma. Br. J. Dis. Chest *75:* 410–412 (1981).

31 Conradi, S.; Ronnevi, L.-O.; Nise, G.; Vesterberg, O.: Long-time penicillamine-treatment in amyotrophic lateral sclerosis with parallel determination of lead in blood, plasma and urine. Acta neurol. *65:* 203–211 (1982).

32 Johnsson, E.A.; Kanerva, L.; Niemi, K.-M.; Lakomaa, E.L.: Generalized argyria with low ceruloplasmin and cupper levels in the serum. A case report with clinical and microscopical findings and a trial of penicillamine treatment. Clin. exp. Dermatol. *7:* 169–176 (1982).

33 Klamer, B.; Kimura, E.T.; Makstenieks, M.: Effects of oral cysteine, penicillamine and N-acetyl-penicillamine on adjuvant arthritis in rats. Pharmacology *1:* 283–287 (1968).

34 Arrigoni-Martelli, E.; Bramm, E.; Huskisson, E.C.; Willoughy, D.A.; Dieppe, P.A.: Pertussis vaccine oedema: an experimental model for the action of penicillamine-like drugs. Agents Actions *6:* 613–616 (1976).

35 Chou, T.; Hill, E.J.; Pathode, R.; Le Quire, V.; Roelofs, R.; Park, J.H.: Penicillamine treatment of hereditary avian muscular dystrophy. Proc. R. Soc. Med. *70:* suppl. 3, pp. 89–93 (1977).

36 Hunneyball, I.M.; Stewart, G.A.; Stanworth, D.R.: Effect of *D*-(–)-penicillamine on chronic experimental arthritis in rabbits. Ann. rheum. Dis. *36:* 378–380 (1977).

37 Savage, A.; Hinton, C.; Tribe, C.R.: Experimental murine amyloidosis. II. Effect of penicillamine therapy. Br. J. exp. Path. *61:* 471–473 (1980).

38 Alley, M.C.; Killiam, E.K.; Fisher, G.L.: The influence of *D*-penicillamine treatment upon seizure activity and trace metal status in the Senegalese baboon, *Papio papio.* J. Pharmac. exp. Ther. *217:* 138–146 (1981).

39 Harris, G.; Chandler, P.M.: Prolonged survival of NZB/NZW female mice treated with oral pyritinol (pyrithioxine); in Maini, Berry, Modulation of autoimmunity and disease, 122–133 (Praeger, 1981).

40 Kerwar, S.S.; Sloboda, A.E.; Birnbaum, J.E.; Oronsky, A.L.: Studies on the effect of *D*-penicillamine on type II collagen-induced polyarthritis. J. Rheumatol. *8:* suppl. 7, pp. 84–88 (1981).

41 Tryfiates, G.P.: Control of tumor growth by pyridoxine restriction or treatment with an antivitamin agent. Cancer Detect. Prevent *4:* 159–164 (1981).

42 Hølund, B.; : 51–55 (1982).

43 Honna, T.; Nakayama, Y.: *D*-Penicillamine-induced enhancement of the delayed hypersensitivity reaction in guinea pigs. Ann. rheum. Dis. *41:* 90–92 (1982).

44 Dixon, A.St.J.; Davies, J.; Dormandy, T.L.; Hamilton, E.B.D.; Holt, P.J.L.; Mason, R.M.; Thompson, M.; Weber, J.C.P.; Zutshi, D.W.: Synthetic *D*(–)-penicillamine in rheumatoid arthritis. Double-blind controlled study of high and low dosage regimen. Ann. rheum. Dis. *34:* 416–421 (1975).

45 Jaffe, I.A.: The technique of penicillamine administration in rheumatoid arthritis. Arthritis Rheum. *18:* 513–514 (1975).

46 Baum, J.: The use of penicillamine in the treatment of rheumatoid arthritis and scleroderma. Scand. J. Rheumatol., suppl. 28, pp. 65–70 (1979).

47 Kean, W.F.; Dwosh, I.L.; Anastassiades, T.P.; Ford, P.M.; Kelly, H.G.: The toxicity pattern of *D*-penicillamine therapy. Arthritis Rheum. *23:* 158–164 (1980).

48 Stein, H.B.; Patterson, A.C.; Offer, R.C.; Atkins, C.J.; Teufel, A.; Robinson, H.S.: Adverse effects of *D*-penicillamine in rheumatoid arthritis. Ann. intern. Med. *92:* 24–29 (1980).

49 Dawkins, R.L.; Zilko, P.J.; Carrano, J.; Garlepp, M.J.; McDonald, B.L.: Immunobiology of *D*-penicillamine. J. Rheumatol. *8:* suppl. 7, pp. 56–61 (1981).

50 Epler, G.R.; Snider, G.L.; Gaensler, E.A.; Cathcart, E.S.; Fitzgerald, M.X.; Carrington, C.B.: Bronchiolitis and bronchitis in connective tissue disease. A possible relationship to the use of penicillamine. J. Am. med. Ass. *242:* 528–532 (1979).

51 Kay, A.G.L.: Myelotoxicity of *D*-penicillamine. Ann. rheum. Dis. *38:* 232–236 (1979).

52 Rooney, P.J.; Cleland, J.: Successful treatment of *D*-penicillamine-induced breast gigantism with danzol. Br. med. J. *282:* 1627–1628 (1981).

53 Seibold, J.R.; Lynch, C.J.; Medsger, T.A.: Cholestasis associated with *D*-Penicillamine therapy: case report and review of the literature. Arthritis Rheum. *24:* 554–560 (1981).

54 Pool, K.D.; Feit, H.; Kirkpatrick, J.: Penicillamine-induced neuropathy in rheumatoid arthritis. Ann. intern. Med. *95:* 457–458 (1981).

55 Sullivan, A.L.; Burakoff, R.; Weintraub, L.R.: Sideroblastic anemia associated with penicillamine therapy. Archs intern. Med. *141:* 1713–1714 (1981).

56 Rothschild, B.: Pyridoxine deficiency. Archs intern. Med. *142:* 840 (1982).

57 Levy, R.S.; Fisher, M.; Alter, J.N.: Penicillamine: review and cutaneous manifestations. J. Am. Acad. Dermatol. *8:* 548–558 (1983).

58 Hickling, P.; Fuller, J.: Penicillamine causing acute colitis. Br. med. J. *ii:* 367 (1979).

59 Lubach, D.; Marghescu, S.: Yellow-nail-Syndrom durch *d*-Penicillamin. Hautarzt *30:* 547–549 (1979).

60 Munroe, D.D.; Darley, C.R.: Hair; in Fitzpatrick, Eisen, Wolff, Freedberg, Austen, Dermatology in general medicine; 2nd ed., pp. 395–418 (McGraw-Hill, New York 1979).

61 Davies, D.; Lloyd Jones, J.K.: Pulmonary eosinophilia caused penicillamine. Thorax *35:* 957–958 (1980).

62 Camus, P.; Degat, O.R.; Justrabo, E.; Jeannin, L.: *D*-Penicillamine-induced severe pneumonitis. Chest *81:* 376–378 (1982).

63 Gilman, P.A.; Holtzman, N.A.: Acute lymphoblastic leukemia in a patient receiving penicillamine for Wilson's disease. J. Am. med. Ass. *248:* 467–468 (1982).

64 Reid, D.M.; Martynoga, A.G.; Nuki, G.: Reversible gynecomastia associated with *D*-penicillamine in a man with rheumatoid arthritis. Br. med. J. *285:* 1083–1084 (1982).

65 Harpey, J.-P.; Jandon, M.-C.; Clavel, J.-P.; Gallis, A.; Darbois, Y.: Cutis laxa and low serum zink after antenatal exposure to penicillamine. Lancet *ii:* 858 (1983).

66 Panayi, G.S.; Wooley, P.; Batchelor, J.R.: Genetic basis of rheumatoid disease: HLA antigens, disease manifestations and toxic reactions to drugs. Br. med. J. *ii:* 1326–1328 (1978).

67 Wooley, P.H.; Griffin, J.; Panayi, G.S.; Batchelor, J.R.; Welsh, K.I.; Gibson, T.J.: HLA-DR antigens and toxic reaction to sodium aurothiomalate and *D*-penicillamine in patients with rheumatoid arthritis. New Engl. J. Med. *303:* 300–302 (1980).

68 Bardin, T.; Dryll, A.; Debeyre, N.; Ruckewaert, A.; Legrand, L.; Marcelli, A.; Dausset, J.: HLA system and side effects of gold salts and *D*-penicillamine treatment of rheumatoid arthritis. Ann. rheum. Dis. *41:* 599–601 (1982).
69 Zilko, P.J.: Discussion. J. Rheumatol. *8:* suppl. 7, p. 173 (1981).
70 Panayi, G.S.; Huston, G.; Shah, R.R.; Mitchell, S.C.; Idle, J.R.; Smith, S.L.; Waring, R.H.: Deficient sulphoxidation status and *D*-penicillamine toxicity. Lancet *i:* 414 (1983).
71 Kean, W.F.; Lock, C.J.L.; Howard-Lock, H.E.; Buchanan, W.W.: Prior gold therapy does not influence the adverse effects of *D*-penicillamine in rheumatoid arthritis. Arthritis Rheum. *25:* 917–922 (1982).
72 Smith, P.J.; Swinburn, W.R.; Swinson, D.R.; Stewart, I.M.: Influence of previous gold toxicity on subsequent development of penicillamine toxicity. Br. med. J. *285:* 595–596 (1982).
73 Miehlke, K.; Jentsch, D.: Der heutige Stand der *D*-Penicillamin-Therapie der chronischen Polyarthritis. Therapiewoche *36:* 3072–3081 (1973).
74 Ott, V.R.; Schmidt, K.L.: Die Behandlung mit *D*-Penicillamin bei rheumatoider Arthritis. Internist *15:* 328–335 (1974).
75 Bálint, G.; Szobor, A.; Temesvári, P.; Zahumensky, Z.; Bozsóky, S.: Myasthenia gravis developed under *D*-penicillamine treatment. Scand. J. Rheumatol., suppl. 8, abstract 21–12 (1975).
76 Bucknall, R.C.; Dixon, A.St.J.; Glick, E.N.; Woodland, J.; Zutshi, D.W.: Myasthenia gravis associated with penicillamine treatment for rheumatoid arthritis. Br. med. J. *i:* 600–602 (1975).
77 Czlonkowska, A.: Myasthenia syndrome during penicillamine treatment. Br. med. J. *ii:* 726–727 (1975).
78 Delrieu, F.; Menkes, C.J.; Sainte-Croix, A.; Babinet, P.; Chesneau, A.M.; Delbarre, F.: Myasthenie et thyroïdite auto-immune au cours d'une polyarthrite rhumatoïde traitée par la *D*-pénicillamine. Nouv. Presse méd. *4:* 2890 (1975).
79 Dawkins, R.L.; Zilko, P.J.; Owen, E.T.: Penicillamine therapy, antistriational antibody, and myasthenia gravis. Br. med. J. *ii:* 759–760 (1975).
80 Schmidt, D.; Kommerell, G.: Okuläre Myasthenie durch *D*-Penicillamin-Behandlung. Klin. Mbl. Augenheilk. *168:* 409–413 (1976).
81 Seitz, D.; Hopf, H.C.; Janzen, R.W.C.; Meyer, W.: Penicillamine-induced myasthenia in chronic rheumatoid arthritis. Dt. med. Wschr. *101:* 1153–1158 (1976).
82 Bucknall, R.C.: Myasthenia associated with *D*-penicillamine therapy in rheumatoid arthritis. Proc. R. Soc. Med. *70:* suppl. 3, pp. 114–117 (1977).
83 Gordon, R.A.; Burnside, J.W.: *D*-Penicillamine-induced myasthenia gravis in rheumatoid arthritis. Ann. intern. Med. *87:* 578–579 (1977).
84 Verret, J.M.; Lignac, N.; Kahn, M.F.: Syndrome myasthénique au cours d'un traitement par la *d*-pénicillamine. Un nouveau cas. Annls Méd int. *128:* 557–560 (1977).
85 Verbraeken, F.J.; Gabriel, P.; Wille, C.: Syndrome myasthénique après traitement peroral à la pénicillamine. Ophthalmologica, Basel *177:* 88–91 (1978).
86 Rosenberger, K.: Myasthenische Reaktionen unter Penicillamin-Behandlung. Medsche Welt, Stuttg. *29:* 976–978 (1978).
87 Russell, A.S.; Lindstrom, J.M.: Penicillamine-induced myasthenia gravis associated with antibodies to acetylcholine receptor. Neurology, Minneap. *28:* 847–849 (1978).

88 Vincent, A.; Newsom-Davis, J.; Martin, V.: Anti-acetylcholine receptor antibodies in *D*-penicillamine-associated myasthenia gravis. Lancet *i:* 1254 (1978).

89 Froelich, C.J.; Hashimoto, F.; Searles, R.P.; Bankhurst, A.D.: *D*-penicillamine-induced myasthenia gravis in rheumatoid arthritis. J. Rheumatol. *6:* 237–239 (1979).

90 Keesey, J.; Novom, S.: HLA antigens in penicillamine-induced myasthenia gravis. Neurology, Minneap. *29:* 528–529 (1979).

91 Sundström, W.R.; Schuma, A.A.: Penicillamine-induced myasthenia gravis. Arthritis Rheum. *22:* 197–198 (1979).

92 Albers, J.W.; Hodach, R.J.; Kimmel, D.W.; Treacy, W.L.: Penicillamine-associated myasthenia gravis. Neurology, Minneap. *30:* 1246–1250 (1980).

93 Blanlœil, Y.; Baron, D.; Nicolas, F.: Syndrome myasthénique induit par la *D*-pénicillamine. Danger de la curarisation. Nouv. Presse méd. *9:* 3695–3696 (1980).

94 Heyn, J.: Penicillamin-induceret myasthenia gravis. Ugeskr. Læg. *142:* 1928–1929 (1980).

95 Rousseau, J.J.; Dieudonné, L.G.: Syndrome myasthénique secondaire à l'administration de *d*-pénicillamine. Acta neurol. psychiat. belg. *80:* 165–173 (1980).

96 Torres, C.F.; Griggs, R.C.; Baum, J.; Penn, A.S.: Penicillamine-induced myasthenia gravis in progressive systemic sclerosis. Arthritis Rheum. *23:* 505–508 (1980).

97 Bocanegra, T.S.; Espinoza, L.R.; Vasey, F.B.; Germain, B.F.; Jaffe, I.A.; Penn, A.S.: Acetylcholine receptor antibodies in penicillamine-induced myasthenia gravis. J. Am. med. Ass. *246:* 1901 (1981).

98 Lang, A.E.; Humphrey, J.G.; Gordon, D.A.: Plasma exchange therapy for severe penicillamine-induced myasthenia gravis. J. Rheumatol. *8:* 303–307 (1981).

99 Rodat, O.; Hamelin, J.-P.; Rossard, A.; Cottin, S.; Cler, J.-M.; Rodat, G.; Lemouroux, P.: Syndromes myasthéniques induits par la *D*-pénicillamine au cours de la polyarthrite rheumatoïde. Deux observations. Nouv. Presse méd. *10:* 1645–1648 (1981).

100 Weinzierl, M.; Kruis, W.; Eisenburg, J.: Myasthenie-Syndrom unter *D*-Penicillamin-Therapie bei primär-biliärer Zirrhose. Internist *22:* 93–95 (1981).

101 Wysocka, K.; Fabian, F.; Listewnik, M.: Myasthenia gravis as a complication of *D*-penicillamine therapy in rheumatoid arthritis. J. Rheumatol. *40:* 135–137 (1981).

102 Essigman, W.K.: Multiple side effects of penicillamine therapy in one patient with rheumatoid arthritis. Ann. rheum. Dis. *41:* 617–620 (1982).

103 Fawcett, P.R.W.; McLachlan, S.M.; Nicholson, L.V.B.; Argov, Z.; Mastaglia, F.: *D*-Penicillamine-associated myasthenia gravis: immunological and electrophysiological studies. Muscle Nerve *5:* 328–334 (1982).

104 Gietka, A.: Miastenia rzekomoporázna w nastepstwie leczenia penicylamina reumatoidalnego zapalenia stawów. Reumatologia *XX:* 66–67 (1982).

105 Vincent, A.; Newson-Davis, J.: Acetylcholine receptor antibody characteristics in myasthenia gravis. II. Patients with penicillamine-induced myasthenia or idiopathic myasthenia of recent onset. Clin. exp. Immunol. *49:* 266–272 (1982).

106a Woimant, F.; Benacin, L.; Delauche, M.C.; Haguenau, M.; Pepin, B.: Syndrome myasténique induit par la *D*-pénicillamine. Evolution du taux sérique des anticorps anti-récepteurs d'acétylcholine. Nouv. Presse méd. *11:* 1807–1808 (1982).

106b Delamere, J.P.; Jobson, S.; Mackintosh, L.P.; Wells, L.; Walton, K.W.: Penicillamine-induced myasthenia gravis in rheumatoid arthritis: its clinical and genetic features. Ann. rheum. Dis. *42:* 500–504 (1983).

107 Garlepp, M.J.; Dawkins, R.L.; Christiansen, F.T.: HLA antigens and acethylcholine receptor antibodies in penicillamine induced myasthenia gravis. Br. med. J. *286:* 338–340 (1983).

108 Smith, C.I.E.; Hammarström, L.; Matell, G.; Nilsson, B.Y.: Role of penicillamine for the induction of myasthenia gravis. Eur. Neurol. *22:* 272–282 (1983).

109 Bucknall, R.C.; Balint, G.; Dawkins, R.L.: Myasthenia associated with *D*-penicillamine therapy in rheumatoid arthritis. Scand. J. Rheumatol., suppl. 28, pp. 91–93 (1979).

110 Storm-Mathisen, A.: Myasthenia gravis: a clinical study with special references to prevalence and prognosis, chapt. 4, p. 58 (Aschehoug, Oslo 1968).

111 Osserman, K.E.: Myasthenia gravis, chapt. 18, p. 263 (Grune & Stratton, New York 1968).

112 Simpson, J.A.: Myasthenia gravis as an autoimmune disease: clinical aspects. Ann. N.Y. Acad. Sci. *135:* 506 (1966).

113 Dawkins, R.L.; Garlepp, M.J.; McDonald, B.L.; Williamson, J.; Zilko, P.J.; Carrano, J.: Myasthenia gravis and *D*-penicillamine. J. Rheumatol. *8:* suppl. 7, pp. 169–172 (1981).

114 Masters, C.L.; Dawkins, R.L.; Zilko, P.J.; Simpson, J.A.; Leedman, R.J.: Penicillamine-associated myasthenia gravis, antiacethylcholine receptor and antistriational antibodies. Am. J. Med. *63:* 691 (1977).

115 Garlepp, M.J.H.; Kay, P.H.; Dawkins, R.L.; Backnall, R.C.; Kemp, A.: Cross-reactivity of anti-acethylcholine receptor autoantibodies. Muscle Nerve *4:* 282–288 (1981).

116 Vincent, A.; Newson-Davis, J.: HLA antigens in penicillamine induced myasthenia gravis. Br. med. J. *286:* 893 (1983).

117 Garlepp, M.J.; Dawkins, R.L.; Christiansen, F.T.: HLA antigens and acetylcholine receptor antibodies in penicillamine induced myasthenia gravis. Br. med. J. *286:* 1442–1443 (1983).

118 Smith, C.I.E.; Aarli, J.A.; Hammarström, L.; Persson, M.A.A.: IgG subclass distribution of myasthenia gravis thymoma associated muscle antibodies. Neurology (in press).

119 Jacobus, D.; Bokelman, D.L.; Majka, J.A.: *D*-Penicillamine in the monkey; in Munthe, Penicillamine research in rheumatic disease, p. 25 (Fabritius & Sønner, Oslo 1976).

120 Pirskanen, R.; Tiilikainen, A.; Hokkanen, E.: Histocompatibility antigens associated with myasthenia gravis. Ann. clin. Res. *4:* 304–306 (1972).

121 Möller, E.; Hammarström, L.; Smith, C.I.E.; Matell, G.: HL-A8 and LD-8a in patients with myasthenia gravis. Tissue Antigens *7:* 39–44 (1976).

122 Dawkins, R.L.; Christiansen, F.T.; Kay, P.H.; Garlepp, M.; McCluskey, J.; Hollingsworth, P.N.; Zilko, P.J.: Disease associations with complotypes, supratypes and haplotypes. Immunol. Rev. *70:* 5–22 (1983).

123 Aldrich, M.S.; Young, I.K.; Sanders, D.B.: Effect of *D*-penicillamine on neuromuscular transmission in rats. Muscle Nerve *2:* 180–185 (1979).

124 Burres, S.A.; Richman, D.P.; Crayton, J.W.; Arnason, B.G.W.: Penicillamine-induced myasthenic responses in the guinea pig. Muscle Nerve *2:* 186–190 (1979).

125 McVicker, J.H.; Lava, N.S.; Mittag, T.W.; Ringel, S.P.: *D*-penicillamine-induced neuromuscular disease in guinea pigs. Expl. Neurol. *76:* 46–57 (1982).

126 Atcheson, S.G.; Ward, J.R.: Ptosis and weakness after start of *D*-penicillamine therapy. Ann. intern. Med. *89:* 939–940 (1978).

127 Jaffe, I.A.: Penicillamine in rheumatoid arthritis. Clinical pharmacology and biochemical properties. Scand. J. Rheumatol., suppl. 28, p. 58 (1979).

128 Bever, T.C.; Chang, H.W.; Penn, A.S.; Jaffe, I.A.; Bock, E.: Penicillamine-induced myasthenia gravis: Effects of penicillamine on acetylcholine receptor. Neurology, Minneap. *32:* 1077–1082 (1982).

129 Jaffe, I.A.: Induction of autoimmune syndromes by penicillamine therapy in rheumatoid arthritis and other diseases. Springer Semin. Immunopathol. *4:* 193–207 (1981).

130 Yung, C.W.; Hambrick, G.W.: *D*-Penicillamine-induced pemphigus syndrome. J. Am. Acad. Dermatol. *6:* 317–324 (1982).

131 Degos, R.; Touraine, R.; Beläich, S.; Revuz, J.: Pemphigus chez un malade traité par pénicillamine pour maladie de Wilson. Bull. Soc. fr. Derm. Syph. *76:* 751–753 (1969).

132 Hewitt, J.; Lessana-Leibowitch, M.; Beneveniste, M.; Saporta, L.: Un cas de pemphigus induit par la *D*-pénicillamine. Le pemphigus iatrogène existe-t-il. Annls Méd. int. *122:* 1003–1009 (1971).

133 Kuffer, R.; Noble, J.P.: Stomatite de la *D*-pénicillamine. Revue Stomat. Chir. maxillo-fac. *74:* 309–320 (1973).

134 Benveniste, M.; Crouzet, J.; Homberg, J.C.; Lessana, M.; Camus, J.P.; Hevitt, J.: Pemphigus induits par la *D*-pénicillamine dans la polyarthrite rhumatoide. Nouv. Presse méd. *4:* 3125–3128 (1975).

135 Cairns, E.J.: Penicillamine-induced pemphigus. Proc. R. Soc. Med. *69:* 384 (1976).

136 Colliard, H.; Saurat, J.H.: Pemphigus induit par la penicillamine. Revue Stomat. Chir. maxillo-fac. *77:* 741–746 (1976).

137 Tan, S.G.; Rowell, N.R.: Pemphigus-like syndrome induced by *D*-penicillamine. Br. J. Derm. *95:* 99–100 (1976).

138 Davies, M.G.; Holt, P.: Pemphigus in a patient treated with penicillamine for generalized morphea. Archs Derm. *112:* 1308–1309 (1976).

139 Marsden, R.A.; Ryan, T.J.; Vanhegan, R.I.; Walshe, M.; Hill, H.; Mowat, A.: Pemphigus foliaceus induced by penicillamine. Br. med. J. *ii:* 1423–1424 (1976).

140 From, E.; Frederiksen, P.: Pemphigus vulgaris following *D*-penicillamine. Dermatologica *152:* 358–362 (1976).

141 Scherak, O.; Kolarz, G.; Molubar, K.: Pemphigus erythematosus-like rash in a patient on penicillamine. Br. med. J. *i:* 838 (1977).

142 Kristensen, J.K.; Wadskov, S.: Penicillamine-induced pemphigus foliaceus. Acta derm.-vener., Stockh. *57:* 69–71 (1977).

143 Stewart, W.M.; Lauret, P.; Boullie, M.C.; Thomine, E.; Avenel, M.: A propos de deux cas d'accidents bulleux, dont un cas de pemphigus, dus à la pénicillamine. Annls Derm. Vénér. *104:* 542–548 (1977).

144 Marsden, R.A.; Dawber, R.P.; Milliard, P.R.: Herpetiform pemphigus induced by penicillamine. Br. J. Derm. *97:* 451–452 (1977).

145 Sparrow, G.P.: Penicillamine pemphigus and the nephrotic syndrome occurring simultaneously. Br. J. Derm. *98:* 103–105 (1978).

146 Christoph, R.; Genth, E.; Grussendorf, E.I.: Pemphigus syndrom bei *D*-penicillamin-behandelter rheumatoider arthritis. Medsche Welt, Stuttg. *29:* 1761–1763 (1978).

147 Thorvaldsen, J.: Two cases of penicillamine-induced pemphigus erythematosus. Dermatologica *159:* 167–170 (1979).

148 Delcambre, B.; Bergoend, H.; Defrance, D.: Le pemphigus induit par la *D*-pénicillamine au cours du traitement de la polyarthrite rhumatoïde. Lille méd. *24:* 283–286 (1979).

149 Trau, H.; Schewach-Millet, M.; Gold, I.; Feinstein, A.; Horowitz, I.; Kaplinsky, N.: Penicillamine-induced pemphigus. Archs Derm. *116:* 721–722 (1980).

150 Marsden, R.A.; Hill, H.; Morvat, A.G.; Walshe, M.; Vanhegan, R.I.; Ryan, T.J.: Penicillamine-induced pemphigus. Proc. R. Soc. Med. *70:* 103–108 (1977).

151 Kennedy, C.; Hodge, L.; Sanderson, K.V.: Skin changes casued by *D*-penicillamine treatment of arthritis. Report of three cases with immunological findings. Clin. exp. Dermatol. *3:* 107–116 (1978).

152 Santa Cruz, D.J.; Marcus, M.D.; Prioleau, P.G.; Uitto, J.: Pemphigus-like lesions induced by *D*-penicillamine. Analysis of clinical, histopathological and immunofluorescence features in 34 cases. Am. J. Dermatopathol. *3:* 85–92 (1981).

153 Barety, M.; Ortonne, J.P.; Chichmanian, R.M.; Lapalus, P.; Savini, E.C.: Pemphigus et traitement par la *D*-pénicillamine. Thérapie *37:* 471–474 (1982).

154 Zone, J.; Ward, J.; Boyce, E.; Schupbach, C.: Penicillamine-induced pemphigus. J. Am. med. Ass. *247:* 2705–2707 (1982).

155 Namba, T.; Brunner, N.G.; Grob, D.: Association of myasthenia gravis with pemphigus vulgaris, candida albicans infection, polymyositis and myocarditis. J. neurol. Sci. *20:* 231–242 (1973).

156 Maize, J.C.; Dobson, R.L.; Provost, T.T.: Pemphigus and myasthenia gravis. Archs Derm. *111:* 1334–1338 (1975).

157 Imamura, S.; Takigawa, M.; Ikai, K.; Yoshinaga, H.; Yamada, M.: Pemphigus foliaceus, myasthenia gravis, thymoma and red cell aplasia, A case report and a study on 38 patients with myasthenia gravis. Clin. exp. Dermatol. *3:* 285–291 (1978).

158 Rapaport, R.J.; Kozin, F.; Mackel, S.E.; Jordon, R.E.: Cutaneous vascular immunofluorescence in rheumatoid arthritis. Correlation with circulating immune complexes and vasculitis. Am. J. Med. *68:* 325–231 (1980).

159 Schuppli, R.: Zur Frage der Abgrenzung des Lyell-Syndroms. Hautarzt *18:* 518–521 (1969).

160 Falk, E.S.: Pemphigus foliaceus in a patient with rheumatoid arthritis and Sjörgen's syndrome. A case report. Dermatologica *158:* 348–354 (1979).

161 Troy, J.L.; Silvers, D.N.; Grossman, M.E.; Jaffe, I.A.: Penicillamine-associated pemphigus: Is it really pemphigus? J. Am. Acad. Dermatol. *4:* 547–555 (1981).

162 Ruocco, V.; de Luca, M.; Pisani, M.; de Angelis, E.; Vitale, O.; Astarita, C.: Pemphigus provoked by *D*(–)-penicillamine. An experimental approach using in vitro tissue cultures. Dermatologica *164:* 236–248 (1982).

163 Katz, S.I.; Dahl, M.V.; Penneys, N.; Trapani, R.J.; Rogentine, N.: HL-A antigens in pemphigus. Archs Derm. *108:* 53–55 (1973).

164 Krain, L.S.; Teresaki, P.I.; Newcomer, V.D.; Mickey, M.R.: Increased frequency of HL-A 10 in pemphigus vulgaris. Archs Derm. *108:* 803–805 (1973).

165 Amar, A.; Rubinstein, N.; Hacham-Zadeh, S.; Cohen, T.; Brautbar, C.: Is predisposition to pemphigus vulgaris in Jewish patients mediated by HLA-Dw 10 and DR 4? Tissue Antigens *23:* 17–22 (1984).

166 Doyle, D.R.; McCurley, T.L.; Sergent, J.S.: Fatal polymyositis in *D*-penicillamine-treated rheumatoid arthritis. Ann. intern. Med. *98:* 327–330 (1983).

167 Schraeder, P.L.; Peters, H.A.; Dahl, D.S.: Polymyositis and penicillamine. Archs Neurol., Chicago *27:* 456–457 (1972).

168 Bettendorf, U.; Neuhaus, R.: Penicillamin-induzierte Polymyositis. Dt. med. Wschr. *99:* 2522–2524 (1974).

169 Nishikai, M.; Funatsu, Y.; Homma, M.: Monoclonal gammopathy, penicillamine-induced polymyositis and systemic sclerosis. Archs Derm. *110:* 253–255 (1974).
170 Cucher, B.G.; Goldman, A.L.: *D*-Penicillamine-induced polymyositis in rheumatoid arthritis. Ann. intern. Med. *85:* 615–616 (1976).
171 Fernandes, L.; Swinson, D.R.; Hamilton, E.B.D.: Dermatomyositis complicating penicillamine treatment. Ann. rheum. Dis. *36:* 94–95 (1977).
172 Petersen, J.; Halberg, P.; Hojgaard, K.; Lyon, B.B.; Ullman, S.: Penicillamine-induced polymyositis-dermatomyositis. Scand. J. Rheumatol. *7:* 113–117 (1978).
173 Simpson, N.B.; Golding, J.R.: Dermatomyositis induced by penicillamine. Acta derm.-vener., Stockh. *59:* 543–544 (1979).
174 Ostensen, M.; Husby, G.; Aarli, J.: Polymyositis with acute myolysis in a patient with rheumatoid arthritis treated with penicillamine and ampicillin. Arthritis Rheum. *23:* 375–377 (1980).
175 Wojnarowska, F.: Dermatomyositis induced by penicillamine. J. soc. Med. *73:* 884–886 (1980).
176 Schlumpf, U.; Bussman, H.U.; Jerusalem, F.: Myositis bei chronischer Polyarthritis unter *D*-Penicillamin, medikamentös induziert? Schweiz. med. Wschr. *111:* 29–35 (1981).
177 Morgan, J.G.; McGuire, J.L.; Ochoa, J.: Penicillamine-induced myositis in rheumatoid arthritis. Muscle Nerve *4:* 137–140 (1981).
178 Marty-Double, C.H.; Pages, M.; Pages, A.M.; Pellisier, J.; Brousson, A.: Etude ultrastructurale d'une polymyosite induite par la *D*-pénicillamine. Archs Anat. Cytol. path. *28:* 325–328 (1980).
179 Fischer, R.G.; Pennebaker, J.B.: Penicillamine-induced polymyositis in a patient with rheumatoid arthritits. Sth. med. J., Nashville *74:* 1286 (1981).
180 Bohan, A.; Peter, J.B.; Bowman, R.L.; Pearson, C.M.: A computer-assisted analysis of 153 patients with polymyositis and dermatomyositis. Medicine, Baltimore *56:* 255 (1977).
181 Behan, W.M.H.; Behan, P.O.; Doyle, D.: Association of myasthenia gravis and polymyositis with neoplasia, infection and autoimmune disorders. Acta neuropath. *57:* 221–229 (1982).
182 Behan, W.M.H.; Behan, P.O.; Dick, H.A.: HLA-B8 in polymyositis. New Engl. J. Med. *298:* 1260–1261 (1978).
183 Boudin, G.; Pépin, B.; Godeau, P.; Vernaut, J.C.; Gouerou, H.: Lupus erythémateux induit par la pénicillamine au cours d'une maladie de Wilson. Annls Méd. int. *122:* 269–273 (1971).
184 Caille, B.; Harpey, J.P.; Lejeune, C.; Sudre, Y.; Turpin, R.: Syndrome lupique induit par la *D*-pénicillamine au cours d'une maladie de Wilson. Etude clinique d'une observation. Annls Méd. int. *122:* 255–260 (1971).
185 Harpey, Moulias, R.; Goust, J.M.; Berthaux, P.: Syndrome lupique induit par la *D*-pénicillamine au cours d'une maladie de Wilson. Etude immunologique par le test de migration des leucocytes (TML). Annls Méd. int. *122:* 261–267 (1971).
186 Rasmussen, K.: Observations during treatment of cystinuria with *D*-penicillamine. Acta med. scand. *189:* 367–372 (1971).
187 Oliver, I.; Lieberman, N.A.; Vries, A.: Lupus like syndrome induced by penicillamine in cystinuria. J. Am. med. Ass. *220:* 588 (1972).
188 Rimbaud, P.; Mirouze, J.; Mary, P.; Meynadier, J.: Complications dermatologiques au

cours du traitement de la maladie de Wilson par la *D*-pénicillamine. Méd. Chir. Dig. *2:* 3–8 (1973).

189 Crouzet, J.; Camus, J.-P.; Leca, A.-P.; Guillieu, P.; Lièvre, J.A.: Lupus induit par la *D*-pénicillamine au cours du traitement de la polyarthrite rhumatoïde au cours de ce traitement. Annls Méd. int. *125:* 71–79 (1974).

190 Harkcom, T.M.; Conn, D.L.; Holley, K.E.: *D*-Penicillamine and lupus erythematosus-like syndrom. Ann. intern. Med. *89:* 1012 (1978).

191 Appelboom, T.; de Maubeuge, J.; Unger, J.; Famaey, J.P.: Cutaneous lupus induced by penicillamine. Scand. J. Rheumatol. *7:* 64 (1978).

192 Kirby, J.D.; Dieppe, P.A.; Huskisson, E.C.; Smith, B.: *D*-Penicillamine and immune complex deposition. Ann. rheum. Dis. *38:* 344–346 (1979).

193 Walshe, J.M.: Penicillamine and the SLE syndrome. J. Rheumatol. *8:* supp. 7, pp. 155–160 (1981).

194 Chalmers, A.; Thompson, D.; Stein, H.E.; Reid, G.; Patterson, A.C.: Systemic lupus erythematosus during penicillamine therapy for rheumatoid arthritis. Ann. intern. Med. *97:* 659–663 (1982).

195 Fischman, A.S.; Abeles, M.; Zaneth, M.; Weinstein, A.; Rothfield, N.F.: The co-existance of rheumatoid arthritis and systemic lupus erythematosus: a case report and review of the literature. J. Rheumatol. *8:* 405–415 (1981).

196 Camus, J.P.; Homber, J.C.; Crouzet, J.; Mery, C.; Delrieu, F.; Massias, P.; Abuaf, N.: Autoantibody formation in *D*-penicillamine-treated rheumatoid arthritis. J. Rheumatol. *8:* suppl. 7, pp. 80–83 (1981).

197 Hughes, G.R.V.: The diagnosis of systemic lupus erythematosus. Br. J. Haemat. *25:* 409–413 (1973).

198 Reinertsen, J.L.; Klippel, J.H.; Johnson, A.H.; Steinberg, A.D.; Deckler, J.L.; Mann, D.L.: B-lymphocyte alloantigens associated with systemic lupus erythematosus. New Engl. J. Med. *299:* 515–518 (1978).

199 Sternlieb, I.; Bennett, B.; Scheinberg, I.H.: *D*-Penicillamine induced Goodpasture's syndrome. Ann. intern. Med. *92:* 673–676 (1976).

200 Gibson, T.; Burry, H.C.; Ogg, C.: Goodpasture syndrome and *D*-penicillamine. Ann. intern. Med. *84:* 100 (1976).

201 McCormick, J.N.; Wood, P.; Bell, D.: Penicillamine-induced Goodpasture's syndrome; in: Munthe, Penicillamine research in rheumatoid Disease, pp. 268–278 (Fabritius & Sønner, Oslo 1976).

202 Matloff, D.S.; Kaplan, M.H.: *D*-Penicillamine-induced Goodpasture like syndrome in primary biliary cirrhosis – successful treatment with plasmapheresis and immunosuppressives. Gastroenterology *78:* 1046–1049 (1980).

203 Gavaghan, T.E.; McNaught, P.J.; Ralston, M.; Hayes, J.M.: Penicillamine-induced 'Goodpasture's syndrome': successful treatment of a fulminant case. Aust. N.Z. J. Med. *11:* 261–265 (1981).

204 Hasselman, M.; Maurier, F.; Lutun, P.; Vetter, J.-M.; Tempe, J.-D.: Syndrome de Goodpastore au cours d'une polyarthrite rhumatoïde traitée par la *D*-pénicillamine. Revue Méd. int. *3:* 237–238 (1982).

205 Swainson, C.P.; Thomson, D.; Short, A.I.K.; Winney, R.J.: Plasma exchange in the successful treatment of drug-induced renal disease Nephron *30:* 244–249 (1982).

206 Rees, A.J.; Peters, D.K.; Compston, D.A.S.; Batchelor, J.R.: Strong association between

HLA-DRW2 and antibody-mediated Goodpasture's syndrome. Lancet *i:* 966–968 (1978).

207 Editorial: Penicillamine nephropathy. Br. med. J. *282:* 761–762 (1981).

208 Lyle, W.H.: Penicillamine. Clin. rheum. Dis. *5:* 569–601 (1979).

209 Epstein, O.; De Villiers, D.; Jain, S.; Potter, B.J.; Thomas, H.C.; Sherlock, S.: Reduction of immune complexes and immunoglobulins induced by *D*-penicillamine in primary biliary cirrhosis. New Engl. J. Med. *300:* 274–278 (1979).

210 Norberg, R.; Wollheim, F.A.; Gedda, P.O.: Circulating protein complexes in *D*-penicillamine therapy of rheumatoid arthritis. Correlation between IgG- and α_1-antitrypsin-IgA complexes and clinical response. Acta med. scand. *208:* 393–396 (1980).

211 Van de Staak, W.J.B.M.; Cotton, D.W.K.; Jonckheer-Venneste, M.M.H.; Boerbooms, A.M.T.H.: Lichenoid eruption following penicillamine. Dermatologica *150:* 372–374 (1975).

212 Seehafer, J.R.; Roger, R.S., III; Fleming, C.R.; Dickson, E.R.: Lichen planus-like lesions caused by penicillamine in primary biliary cirrhosis. Archs Derm. *117:* 140–142 (1981).

213 Graham-Brown, R.A.C.; Sarkany, I.; Sherlock, S.: Lichen planus and primary biliary cirrhosis. Br. J. Derm. *106:* 699–703 (1982).

214 Powel, F.C.; Rogers, R.S., III; Dickson, E.R.: Lichen planus primary biliary cirrhosis and penicillamine. Br. J. Derm. *107:* 616 (1982).

215 Powell, F.C.; Rogers, R.S., III: Primary biliary cirrhosis, penicillamine and lichen planus. Lancet *ii:* 525 (1981).

216 Tan, R.S.-H.: Ulcerative colitis, myasthenia gravis, atypical lichen planus, alopecia areata, vitiligo, Proc. R. Soc. Med. *67:* 195 (1974).

217 Tan, R.S.-H.: Thymoma aquired hypogammaglobulinemia, lichen planus, alopecia areata. Proc. R. Soc. Med. *67:* 196 (1974).

218 Aronson, I.K.; Soltani, K.; Paik, K.-I.; Rubenstein, D.; Lorincz, A.L.: Triad of lichen planus, myasthenia gravis, and thymoma. Archs Derm. *114:* 255–259 (1978).

219 Flamenbaum, H.S.; Safai, B.; Siegal, F.P.; Pahwa, S.: Lichen planus in immunodeficient hosts. J. Am. Acad. Dermatol. *6:* 918–920 (1982).

220 Lowe, N.J.; Cudworth, A.G.; Woodrow, J.C.: HLA antigens in lichen planus. Br. J. Derm. *95:* 169–171 (1976).

221 Saurat, J.H.; Lemarchand, F.; Hors, J.; Nunez-Roldan, A.; Gluckman, E.; Dausset, J.: HLA markers and lymphocytotoxins in lichen planus. Archs Derm. *113:* 1719–1720 (1977).

222 Bertrand, J.L.; Rousset, H.; Queneau, P.; Ollignier, M.: Thyroïdite auto-immune. Une complication rare du traitement à la *D*-pénicillamine. Thérapie *36:* 333–336 (1981).

223 Ahmed, F.; Sumalnop, V.; Spain, D.M.; Tobin, M.S.: Thrombohemolytic thrombocytopenic purpura during penicillamine therapy. Archs intern. Med. *138:* 1292–1293 (1978).

224 Speth, P.A.J.; Boerbooms, A.M.T.; Holdrinet, R.S.G.; Van de Putte, L.B.A.; Meyer, J.W.R.: Thrombatic thrombocytopenic purpura associated with *D*-penicillamine treatment in rheumatoid arthritis. J. Rheumatol. *9:* 812–813 (1982).

225 May, V.; Aristoff, H.; Lecoq, G.: Syndrome de Gougerot-Sjögren induit par la *D*-pénicillamine. A propos d'un cas. Revue Rhum. Mal. ostéo-artic. *44:* 497–501 (1977).

226 Jaffe, I.A.: Penicillamine treatment of rheumatoid arthritis; in Munthe, Penicillamine research in rheumatoid disease, p. 11 (Fabritius & Sønner, Oslo 1976).

227 Van de Stadt, R.J.; Muijsers, A.O.; Henrichs, A.M.A.; van der Korst, J.K.: *D*-Penicillamine3 biochemical, metabolic and pharmacological aspects. Scand. J. Rheumatol., suppl. 28, pp. 13–20 (1979).

228 Zuckner, J.; Ramsey, R.H.; Dorner, R.W.; Gantner, G.E., Jr.: *D*-Penicillamine in rheumatoid arthritis. Arthritis Rheum. *13:* 131–138 (1970).

229 Wernick, R.; Merryman, P.; Jaffe, I.; Ziff, M.: IgG and IgM rheumatoid factors in rheumatoid arthritis. Quantitative response to penicillamine therapy and relationship to disease activity. Arthritis Rheum. *26:* 593–598 (1983).

230 Stanworth, D.R.; Hunneyball, I.M.: Influence of *D*-penicillamine treatment on the humoral immune system. Scand. J. Rheumatol., suppl. 28, pp. 37–46 (1979).

231 Stephens, A.D.; Fenton, J.C.B.: Serum immunoglobulins in *D*-penicillamine-treated cystinurics. Proc. R. Soc. Med. *70,* suppl. 3, pp. 31 (1977).

232 Strickland, G.D.; Leu, M.-L.: Wilson's disease. Clinical and laboratory manifestations in 40 patients. Medicine, Baltimore *54:* 113–137 (1975).

233 Proesmans, W.; Jaeken, J.; Eeckels, R.: *D*-Penicillamine-induced IgA deficiency in Wilson's disease. Lancet *ii:* 804–805 (1976).

234 Hjalmarson, O.; Hanson, L.Å; Nilsson, L.-Å.: IgA deficiency during *D*-penicillamine treatment. Br. med. J. *6073:* 549 (1977).

235 Michel, F.-B.; Bousquet, J.; Robinet-Levy, M.; Mary, P.: Déficit immunitaire lors d'un traitement par *D*-pénicillamine. Nouv. Presse méd. *6:* 3546–3547 (1977).

236 Stanworth, D.R.; Johns, P.; Williamson, N.; Shadforth, M.; Felix-Davies, D.; Thompson, R.: Drug-induced IgA deficiency in rheumatoid arthritis. Lancet *i:* 1001–1002 (1977).

237 Götze, H.: *D*-Penicillamin-induzierter IgA-Mangel. Klin. Pädiat. *191:* 433–435 (1979).

238 Johns, P.; Felix-Davies, D.D.; Hawkins, C.F.; Macintosh, P.; Shadforth, M.F.; Stanworth, D.R.; Thomson, R.A.; Williamson, N.: IgA deficiency in patients with rheumatoid arthritis treated with *D*-penicillamine or gold. Ann. Rheum. Dis. *37:* 289 (1978).

239 Delamere, J.P.; Grindulis, K.A. and Far, M.: Effects on rheumatoid activity of drug-induced changes in serum immunoglobulins, particularity selective IgA deficiency. Ann. rheum. Dis. *42:* 231 (1983).

240 Mbuyi-Mnamba, J.M.; Stevens, E.; Dequeker, J.: Good response to *D*-penicillamine in IgA-deficient rheumatoid arthritis. Scand. J. Rheumatol. *10:* 31–32 (1981).

241 Hammarström, L.; Axelsson, U.; Gjörkander, J.; Hanson, L.-Å.; Möller, E.; Smith, C.I.E.: Differences in the distribution of HLA antigens in healthy IgA deficient blood donors and in IgA deficient patients with recurrent respiratory tract infections (submitted for publication).

242 Fontana, A.; Joller, H.; Skvaril, F.; Grob, P.: Immunologic abnormalities and HLA antigen frequenices in IgA deficient patients with epilepsi. J. Neurol. Neurosurg. Psychiat. *41:* 593–597 (1978).

243 Hammarström, L.; Smith, C.I.E.: HLA-A,B,C and DR antigens in immunoglobulin A deficiency. Tissue Antigens *21:* 75–79 (1983).

244 Hammarström, L.; Persson, M.A.A.; Smith, C.I.E.: Anti-IgA in selective IgA deficiency: in vitro effects and Ig subclass pattern of human anti-IgA. Scand. J. Immunol. (in press).

245 Bacon, P.A.; Blake, D.R.; Alexander, G.J.M.; Hall, N.D.: Alterations in immunological parameters associated with *D*-penicillamine therapy; in Maine, Berry, Modulation of autoimmunity and disease, pp. 10–15 (Praeger, New York 1981).

246 Chawalinska-Sadowska, H.; Baum, J.: The effect of *D*-penicillamine on polymorphonuclear leucocyte function. J. clin. Invest. *58:* 871–879 (1976).
247 Mellbye, O.J.; Munthe, E.: Effect of penicillamine on complement in vitro and in vivo. Ann. rheum. Dis. *36:* 453–458 (1977).
248 Tobin, M.S.; Altman, K.: Accelerated immune response induced by *D-L* penicillamine. Proc. Soc. exp. Biol. Med. *115:* 225–228 (1964).
249 Altman, K.; Tobin, M.S.: Suppression of the immune response induced by *D-L* penicillamine. Proc. Soc. exp. Biol. Med. *118:* 554–557 (1965).
250 Assem, E.S.K.; Vickers, M.R.: Immunological response to penicillin-allergic patients and in normal subjects. Prost-grad. med. J., suppl., pp. 65–70 (1974).
251 Roath, S.; Wills, R.: The effects of penicillamine on lymphocytes in culture. Post-grad. med. J., suppl., pp. 56–57 (1974).
252 Brandt, L.; Svensson, B.: Effect of penicillamine on peripheral blood lymphocytes in rheumatoid arthritis. Lancet *i:* 394–395 (1975).
253 Schumacher, K.; Maerker-Alzer, G.; Preuss, R.: Effect of *D*-penicillamine on lymphocyte function. Arzneimittel-Forsch. *25:* 603–606 (1975).
254 Kendall, P.A.; Hutchins, D.: The effect of thiol compounds on lymphocytes stimulated in culture. Immunology *35:* 189–201 (1978).
255 Lipsky, P.E.; Ziff, M.: The effect of *D*-penicillamine on mitogen-induced human lymphocyte proliferation: synergistic inhibition by *D*-penicillamine and copper salts. J. Immun. *120:* 1006–1013 (1978).
256 Claesson, M.H.; Sönderstrup Hansen, G.; Tjell, V.: *D*-penicillamine: mitogenic effect on mouse, rat and human spleen lymphocytes. Med. Microbiol. Immunol. *167:* 161–174 (1979).
257 Kosaka, S.: Effects of oral administration of *D*-penicillamine on T-and B-lymphocytes in peripheral blood of rheumatoid patients. Tokoku J. exp. Med. *129:* 233–239 (1979).
258 Room, G.; Roffe, L.; Maini, R.N.: The inhibitory effect of *D*-penicillamine on human lymphocyte cultures stimulated by phytohaemagglutinin, the antagonistic action of *L*-cysteine and synergistic inhibition by copper sulphate. Scand. J. Rheumatol., supp. 28, pp. 47–57 (1979).
259 Feickert, H.F.; Schumacher, K.: Untersuchungen zum Wirkungsmechanismus von *D*-Penicillamin (DPA) auf menschliche Lymphozyten. Arzneimittel-Forsch. *30:* 1480–1483 (1980).
260 Lipsky, P.E.; Ziff, M.: Inhibition of human helper T cell function in vitro by *D*-penicillamine and $CuSO_4$. J. clin. Invest. *65:* 1069–1076 (1980).
261 Binderup, L.; Bramm, E.; Arrigoni-Martelli, E.: *D*-Penicillamine and macrophages: modulation of lymphocyte transformation by concanavalin A. Scand. J. Immunol. *7:* 259–264 (1978).
262 Binderup, L.; Arrigoni-Martelli, E.: ^{14}C-*D*-Penicillamine: uptake and distribution in rat lymphocytes and macrophages. Biochem. Pharmac. *28:* 189–192 (1979).
263 Binderup, L.; Bramm, E.; Arrigoni-Martelli, E.: *D*-Penicillamine in vivo enhances lymphocyte DNA synthesis: role of macrophages. Scand. J. Immunol. *11:* 23–28 (1980).
264 Binderup, L.; Bramm, E.; Arrigoni-Martelli, E.: Effect of *D*-penicillamine in vitro and in vivo on macrophage phagocytosis. Biochem. Pharmac. *29:* 2273–2278 (1980).
265 De Vries, E.; Haasnoot, C.J.P.; Van der Weij, J.P.; Cats, A.: In vitro monocyte-lymphocyte interaction influenced by *d*-penicillamine. Clin. exp. Immunol. *47:* 474–480 (1982).
266 Cunningham, F.M.; Ford-Hutchinson, A.W.; Oliver, A.M.; Smith, M.J.H.; Walker,

J.R.: The effects of *D*-penicillamine and levamisole on leucocyte chemotaxis in the rat. Br. J. Pharmacol. *63:* 119–123 (1978).

267 Mowat, A.G.: Neutrophil chemotaxis in rheumatoid arthritis. Ann. rheum. Dis. *37:* 1–8 (1978).

268 Meacock, S.C.R.; Kitchen, A.; Dawson, W.: Studies on the mode of action of *D*-penicillamine in animal models of inflammation; in Maini, Berry, Modulation of autoimmunity and disease, pp. 115–121 (Praeger, New York 1981).

C.I. Edvard Smith, MD, Department of Clinical Immunology, F 79,
Huddinge University Hospital, S-141 86 Huddinge (Sweden)

Subject Index